STANDARD FIRST AID
AND
PERSONAL SAFETY

The American National Red Cross

AMERICAN RED CROSS

STANDARD FIRST AID AND PERSONAL SAFETY

Prepared by The American
National Red Cross
for the Instruction of
First Aid Classes

First Edition 1973
With 206 Illustrations

**Fourth Printing
December 1975**

DOUBLEDAY & COMPANY, INC.
Garden City, New York

ISBN: 0-385-05848-9 CLOTHBOUND
0-385-05908-6 PAPERBOUND

© 1973 by
The American National Red Cross
All Rights Reserved
Illustrations © 1973 by
The American National Red Cross
Washington, D.C.
Library of Congress Catalog Card No. 73-76726
Printed in the United States of America

PREFACE

Since 1910, the American National Red Cross has provided first aid instruction to the American public.

The First Aid Program of the American National Red Cross, for which this book is a teaching text, stems from the congressional charter provision that the organization shall devise and carry on measures for relieving and preventing suffering.

This textbook is designed for use by the general public to prepare people, through providing them with knowledge and skills, to meet the needs of most situations when emergency first aid care is needed and medical assistance is not excessively delayed. It incorporates personal safety and accident prevention information to acquaint individuals with many causes of accidents so that action can be taken to eliminate or minimize such causes.

To define current remedial procedures for this textbook, the Red Cross has asked the Division of Medical Sciences, National Academy of Sciences-National Research Council, to provide information for developing the content. The Division's assistance ensures the authoritative basis for the course content and provides a channel for extending the first aid recommendations of the medical profession to the American public.

The Red Cross expresses deep appreciation to members of the Ad Hoc Committee for Revision of the Red Cross First Aid Manual, under the chairmanship of Dr. Warren H. Cole, University of Illinois Medical Center, Chicago, Illinois, and to the staff of the Division of Medical Sciences. The Red Cross acknowledges, in particular, the contributions of Dr. Sam F. Seeley, Professional Associate, Division of Medical Sciences, for his technical guidance in developing this textbook prior to his retirement from the National Academy of Sciences. Thanks also are due to Dr. Virginia H. Blocker of Galveston, Texas, for her advice and assistance.

Appreciation for special assistance is also extended to the following Red Cross staff members: Thomas G. Parker, Albert S. Justus, Thomas D. Miller, and C. P. Dail, Jr.

John T. Goetz, director of the American National Red Cross First Aid Program, was responsible for the coordination of materials and the development of this textbook.

The book was illustrated by Angeline V. Culfogienis.

CONTENTS

1

INTRODUCTION TO FIRST AID

I. DEFINITION

First aid is the immediate care given to a person who has been injured or has been suddenly taken ill. It includes self-help and home care if medical assistance is not available or is delayed. It includes well-selected words of encouragement, evidence of willingness to help, and promotion of confidence by demonstration of competence.

II. REASONS FOR FIRST AID

A. First aid knowledge and skill often mean—
1. The difference between life and death
2. The difference between temporary and permanent disability
3. The difference between rapid recovery and long hospitalization

B. First aid training is of value in—
1. Preventing and caring for accidental injury or sudden illness
2. Caring for persons caught in a natural disaster or other catastrophe
3. Equipping individuals to deal with the whole situation, the person, and the injury
4. Distinguishing between what to do and what not to do

C. First aid training is needed because—
1. Statistics show that among persons from age 1 to age 38,

accidents are the leading cause of death, and thereafter they remain one of the leading causes.

    a. The death rate is twice as high among males as females.

    b. The annual cost of medical attention, loss of earning ability due to temporary or permanent impairment, and direct property damage and insurance costs amount to many billions of dollars each year.

    c. Accidents take their toll in pain and suffering, disability, and personal tragedy.

    d. Motor vehicle accidents account for approximately half of all accidental deaths.

2. The concept of massive numbers of casualties has become a reality with the advent of the nuclear age.

3. The pattern of medical care has changed.

4. The growing population and expanding health needs have not been balanced by a proportional increase in numbers of doctors, nurses, and allied health workers.

5. The limitation of *time* in case of an accident or sudden illness may be so critical in terms of *minutes or even seconds* that only a person with first aid knowledge and skills who is on hand has any opportunity of preventing a fatal outcome.

D. First aid training promotes safety awareness in the home, at work, at play, and on streets and highways. In the promotion of such awareness, it is important to closely relate three terms: cause, effect, and prevention.

1. Cause

When in-depth study of an actual or hypothetical accident situation identifies all the causative factors, it becomes possible to determine *what* can be done to eliminate, control, or avoid the hazards.

2. Effect

When analysis carefully considers both immediate and long-range, or permanent, effects of injury or sudden illness, it becomes obvious *why* every possible effort should be taken to eliminate, control, or avoid a situation that is hazardous to oneself or to others.

3. Prevention

A better understanding of the overall accident problem is developed if all the circumstances surrounding various types of accidents are carefully studied. Preventive mea-

sures should include consideration of *how* accident-caus-
ing conditions and activities can be eliminated, controlled,
or avoided.

III. VALUE OF FIRST AID TRAINING

A. Help for others

Through the study of first aid, a person is prepared to assist
others wisely if they are stricken, to give them instruction in
first aid, and to promote among them a reasonable safety
attitude. On a humanitarian basis, there is always an obliga-
tion to assist the stricken and the helpless. There is no greater
satisfaction than that of relieving suffering or saving the life
of a member of your family, a coworker, an acquaintance, or
a stranger.

B. Self-help

In being prepared to help others, the first-aider is better able
to care for himself in case of injury or sudden illness. Even
when his condition is so bad that he is unable to care for
himself, he can direct others in the correct procedures to be
taken in his behalf.

C. Preparation for disaster

First aid training is of particular importance in time of catastrophe, when medical and hospital services are limited or
delayed. Catastrophe may take the form of well-publicized
disasters, such as hurricanes, floods, earthquakes, tornadoes,
and fires. It also may take the form of a single accidental
death, or life-threatening illness. Knowing what to do in an
emergency helps to avoid the panic and disorganized behavior characteristic of unprepared persons at such times.
Knowledge of first aid is a civic responsibility: It not only
helps to save lives and prevent complications from injuries
but also helps in setting up an orderly method of handling
emergency problems according to their priority for treatment
so that the greatest possible good may be accomplished for
the greatest number of people.

IV. GENERAL DIRECTIONS FOR GIVING FIRST AID

As a first-aider, you may encounter a variety of problem situations. Your decisions and actions will vary according to the circumstances that produced the accident or sudden illness, the number of persons involved, the immediate environment, the availability of medical assistance, emergency dressings and equipment, and help from others. You will need to adapt what you have learned to the situation at hand, or to improvise.

Sometimes prompt action is needed to save a life. At other times there is no need for haste, and efforts will be directed toward preventing further injury, obtaining assistance, and reassuring the victim, who may be emotionally upset and apprehensive, as well as in pain.

First aid begins with action, which in itself has a calming effect. If there are multiple injuries or if several persons are hurt, priorities must be set. Enlist the help of bystanders to make telephone calls, to direct traffic, to keep others at a distance if necessary, to position safety flares in case of highway accidents, and perform similar duties. Provide life support to victims with life-threatening injuries, then care for those with less critical injuries.

Telephone, or have someone else telephone, the appropriate authorities regarding an accident. The police department or the highway patrol is a good first contact; but the circumstances surrounding the accident should be a guide as to whom to call. Always have a list of emergency numbers available; if the numbers are not readily available, ask the telephone operator for assistance. Describe the problem, indicate what is being done, and request the assistance needed, such as an ambulance, the fire department, the rescue squad, or utility company personnel. Give your name, the location of the accident, the number of persons involved, and the telephone number where you can be reached. *Do not hang up* the receiver until after the other party hangs up because he may wish to clarify some information.

A. Urgent care

In case of serious injury or sudden illness, while help is being summoned, give *immediate* attention to the following first aid priorities:

1. Effect a prompt rescue. (For example, remove an accident victim from water, from a fire, or from a garage or room containing carbon monoxide, smoke, or noxious fumes.)

2. Ensure that the victim has an open airway and give mouth-to-mouth or mouth-to-nose artificial respiration, if necessary.
3. Control severe bleeding.
4. Give first aid for poisoning, or ingestion of harmful chemicals.

Specific emergencies that require immediate first aid will be discussed fully in appropriate chapters in the text.

B. Additional first aid directions

Once emergency measures have been taken to ensure the victim's safety, the following procedures should be carried out:

1. Do *not* move a victim unless it is necessary for safety reasons. Keep the victim in the position best suited to his condition or injuries; do not let him get up or walk about.
2. Protect the victim from unnecessary manipulation and disturbance.
3. Avoid or overcome chilling by using blankets or covers, if available. If the victim is exposed to cold or dampness, place blankets or additional clothing over and under him.
4. Determine the injuries or cause for sudden illness. After immediate problems are under control—

   a. Find out exactly what happened. Information may be obtained from the victim or from persons who were present and saw the accident, or saw the individual collapse in the case of sudden illness.
   b. Look for an emergency medical identification, such as a card or bracelet, which may provide a clue to the victim's condition.
   c. If the victim is unconscious and has *no* sign of external injury, and if the above methods fail to provide identity, try to obtain proper identification either from papers carried in a billfold or purse, or from bystanders, so that relatives may be notified. (It is advisable to have a witness when searching for identification.)

5. Examine the victim methodically but be guided by the kind of accident or sudden illness and the needs of the situation. Have a reason for what you do.

a. Loosen constricting clothing but do not pull on the victim's belt in case spinal injuries are present.

b. Open or remove clothing if necessary to expose a body part in order to make a more accurate check for injuries. Clothing may be cut away or ripped at the seams, but utmost caution must be used or added injury may result. Do not expose the victim unduly without protective cover, and use discretion if clothing must be removed.

c. Note the victim's general appearance, including skin discoloration, and check all symptoms that may give a clue to the injury or sudden illness.

In the case of a victim with dark skin, change in skin color may be difficult to note. It may then be necessary to depend upon change in the color of the mucous membrane, or inner surface of the lips, mouth, and eyelids.

d. Check the victim's pulse. If you cannot feel it at the wrist, check for a pulse of the carotid artery at the side of his neck.

e. Check to see if the victim is awake, stuporous, or unconscious. Does he respond to questions?

f. If the victim is unconscious, look for evidence of head injury. In a conscious person, look for paralysis of one side of the face or body. See if the victim shows evidence of a recent convulsion. (He may have bitten his tongue, producing a laceration.)

g. Check the expression of the victim's eyes and the size of his pupils.

h. Examine the victim's trunk and limbs for open and closed wounds or for signs of fractures.

i. Check the front of the victim's neck to determine whether he is a laryngectomee. (Most laryngectomees carry a card or other identification stating that they cannot breathe through the nose or mouth.) Do not block the stoma (air inlet) of a laryngectomee when carrying out other first aid, since blockage could cause death from asphyxiation (see chapter 5).

j. If poisoning is suspected, check for stains or burns about the victim's mouth and a source of poisoning nearby, such as pills, medicine bottles, household chemicals, or pesticides.

6. Carry out the indicated first aid:
   a. Apply emergency dressings, bandages, and splints, as indicated.
   b. Do not move the victim unless absolutely necessary.
   c. Plan action according to the nature of the injury or sudden illness, the needs of the situation, and the availability of human and material resources.
   d. Utilize proper first aid measures and specific techniques that, under the circumstances, appear to be reasonably necessary.
   e. Remain in charge until the victim can be turned over to qualified persons (for example, a physician, an ambulance crew, a rescue squad, or a police officer), or until the victim can take care of himself or can be placed in the care of relatives.
   f. Do not attempt to make a diagnosis of any sort or to discuss a victim's condition with bystanders or reporters.
   g. Above all, as a first aid worker, you should know the limits of your capabilities and must make every effort to avoid further injury to the victim in your attempt to provide the best possible emergency first aid care.

2

WOUNDS

I. DEFINITION

A wound is a break in the continuity of the tissues of the body, either internal or external.

A. Classification of wounds

1. Open
   An open wound is a break in the skin or the mucous membrane.
2. Closed
   A closed wound involves injury to underlying tissues without a break in the skin or a mucous membrane.

B. Types of open wounds

1. Abrasions
2. Incisions
3. Lacerations
4. Punctures
5. Avulsions

II. COMMON CAUSES

Wounds usually result from external physical forces. The most common accidents resulting in open wounds are motor vehicle accidents, falls, and mishandling of sharp objects, tools, machinery, and weapons.

III. SYMPTOMS

A. Abrased wounds (Fig. 1)

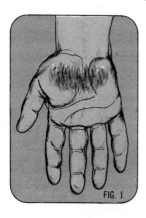

1. The outer layers of the protective skin are damaged. Abrased wounds usually result when the skin is scraped against a hard surface.
2. Bleeding is limited.
3. Danger of contamination and infection exists.

B. Incisions (Fig. 2)

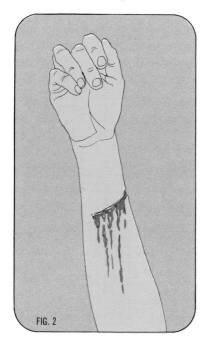

1. An incised wound, or cut, frequently occurs when body tissue is cut on knives, rough edges of metal, broken glass, or other sharp objects.
2. Bleeding may be rapid and heavy.
3. Deep cuts may damage muscles, tendons, and nerves.

C. Lacerations (Fig. 3)

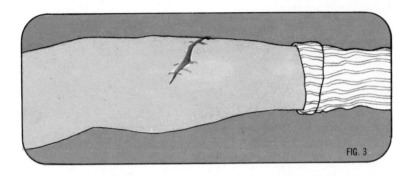

FIG. 3

1. A lacerated wound displays jagged, irregular, or blunt breaking or tearing of the soft tissues, and is usually caused when great force is exerted against the body.
2. Bleeding may be rapid and extensive.
3. Destruction of tissue is greater in a lacerated wound than in a cut.
4. Deep contamination of the wound increases the chance for later infection.

D. Punctures (Fig. 4)

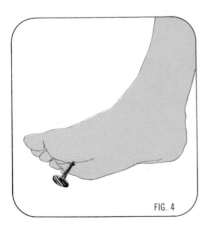

FIG. 4

1. A punctured wound is produced by an object piercing skin layers, creating a small hole in the tissues. Puncture-producing objects include bullets and pointed objects, such as pins, nails, and splinters.
2. External bleeding is usually quite limited.
3. Internal damage may have resulted to the organs, causing internal bleeding.
4. The hazard of infection is increased because the flushing action of external bleeding is limited.
5. Tetanus may develop.

E. Avulsions (Fig. 5)

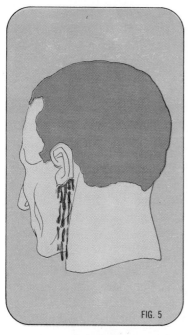

FIG. 5

1. An avulsed wound results when tissue is forcibly separated or torn from the victim's body.
2. An incised wound, a lacerated wound, or both will usually occur when a body part is avulsed.
3. There will be heavy, rapid bleeding.
4. An avulsed body part may be successfully reattached to a victim's body by a surgeon. Send the body part along with the victim to the hospital.
5. Avulsed wounds occur in accidents such as motor vehicle wrecks, gunshots, explosions, animal bites, and other body-crushing injuries.

IV. FIRST AID FOR OPEN WOUNDS

A. Stop the bleeding immediately.

B. Protect the wound from contamination and infection.

C. Provide shock care.

D. Obtain medical attention.

V. FIRST AID FOR SEVERE BLEEDING

A. Need for immediate action

Shock and loss of consciousness in a victim may occur from the rapid loss of as little as a quart of blood. Because it is possible for a victim to bleed to death in a very short period of time, a first-aider should stop any large, rapid loss of blood immediately and treat for shock.

B. Techniques to stop severe bleeding (described in order of preference)

1. Direct pressure

   a. Direct pressure by hand over a dressing is the preferred method for the control of severe bleeding, since it prevents loss of blood from the body without interference with normal blood circulation. In an emergency, in the absence of compresses, the bare hand or fingers may be used, but only until a compress can be applied.

   b. Apply direct pressure by placing the palm of the hand on a dressing directly over the entire area of an open wound on any surface part of the body. In most instances this technique will stop the bleeding (Fig. 6).

   c. A thick pad of cloth held between the hand and the wound helps to control the bleeding by absorbing the blood and allowing it to clot.

   d. Do not disturb blood clots after they have formed within the cloth. If blood soaks through the entire pad without clotting, do not remove the pad, but add additional thick layers of cloth and continue the direct hand pressure even more firmly (Fig. 7).

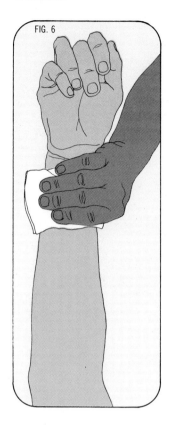

FIG. 6

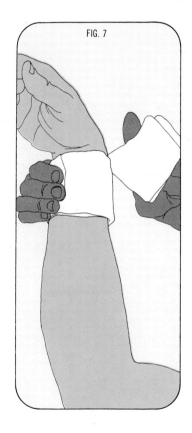

FIG. 7

e. On most parts of the body, a pressure bandage can be placed to hold pads of cloth over a severely bleeding open wound and free the hands of the first-aider for other emergency action.

f. To apply the pressure bandage, place and hold the center of the bandage or strip of cloth directly over the pad on the wound; maintain a steady pull on the bandage to hold the pad firmly in place as you wrap both ends of it around the body part (Figs. 8 and 9),

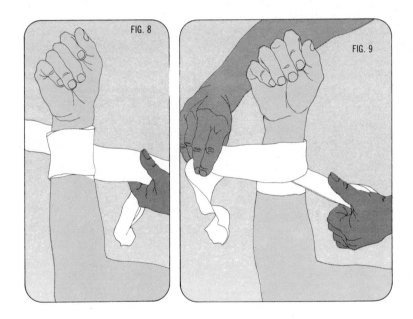

FIG. 8

FIG. 9

and then tie the bandage with the knot directly over the pad (Fig. 10).

2. Elevation

a. Unless there is evidence of a fracture, a severely bleeding open wound of the hand, neck, arm, or leg should

be elevated; that is, the injured part of the body should
be raised above the level of the victim's heart (Fig. 11).

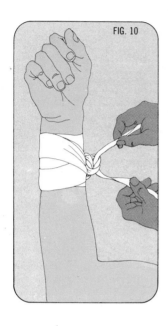

FIG. 10

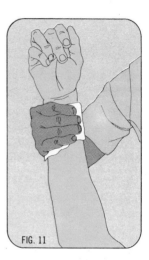

FIG. 11

    b. Elevation uses the force of gravity to help reduce blood
       pressure in the injured area and thus aids in slowing
       down the loss of blood through the wound. However,
       direct pressure on a thick pad over the wound must be
       continued.

3. Pressure on the supplying artery

    a. If severe bleeding from an open wound of the arm or
       leg does not stop after the application of direct pres-
       sure plus elevation, the pressure point technique may
       be required.

    b. Use of the pressure point technique temporarily com-
       presses the main artery (which supplies blood to the

affected limb) against the underlying bone and nearby
tissues (Fig. 12). The technique also stops circulation
within the limb.

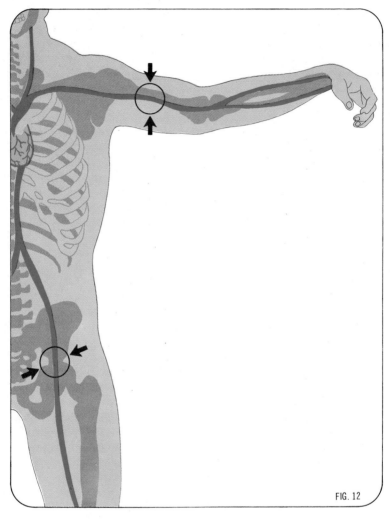

FIG. 12

   c. If the use of a pressure point should be necessary, *do
     not substitute* its use for direct pressure and elevation,
     but use the pressure point in addition to those tech-
     niques.

   d. As a rule, do not use a pressure point in conjunction
     with direct pressure and elevation any longer than

necessary to stop the bleeding. Be prepared, however, to reapply pressure at a pressure point if bleeding recurs.

e. Use the brachial artery for the control of severe bleeding from an open arm wound.

   (1) Apply pressure over the brachial artery, forcing it against the arm bone. The pressure point is located on the inside of the arm in the groove between the biceps and the triceps, about midway between the armpit and the elbow.

   (2) To apply pressure on the brachial artery, grasp the middle of the victim's upper arm, your thumb on the outside of his arm and your other fingers on the inside. Press your fingers toward your thumb to create an inward force from opposite sides of the arm. Use the flat, inside surface of your fingers, not your fingertips. This pressure inward holds and closes the artery by compressing it against the arm bone (Figs. 13A and 13B).

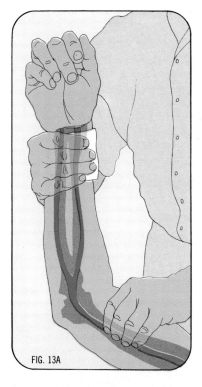
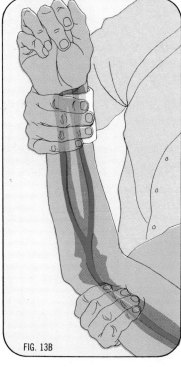

FIG. 13A   FIG. 13B

f. Use the femoral artery for the control of severe bleeding from an open leg wound.

   (1) Apply pressure on the femoral artery by forcing the artery against the pelvic bone. The pressure point is located on the front, center part of the diagonally slanted "hinge" of the leg, in the crease of the groin area, where the artery crosses the pelvic bone on its way to the leg.

   (2) To apply pressure on the femoral artery, position the victim flat on his back, if possible, and place the heel of your hand directly over the pressure point. Then lean forward over your straightened arm to apply the amount of pressure needed to close the artery. Keep your arm straight to prevent arm tension and muscular strain while you apply this technique (Fig. 14). If bleeding is not controlled, it may be necessary to compress directly over the artery with the flat of the fingertips and apply additional pressure over the fingertips with the heel of the other hand.

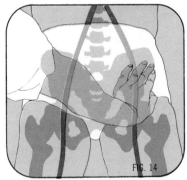

FIG. 14

4. Tourniquet

The use of a tourniquet is dangerous, and the tourniquet should be used only for a severe, life-threatening hemorrhage that cannot be controlled by other means. Tourniquets are used far too often and are rarely required; they should not be used except in critical emergencies when direct pressure on appropriate pressure points fails to stop bleeding. *The decision to apply a tourniquet is in reality a decision to risk sacrifice of a limb in order to save life.*

Once a tourniquet is applied, care by a physician is imperative. (NOTE. A tourniquet should be at least 2 inches wide.)

a. Place the tourniquet just above the wound; do not allow it to touch the wound edges. If the wound is in a joint area or just below, place the tourniquet immediately above the joint.

b. Wrap the tourniquet band tightly around the limb twice and tie a half knot (Fig. 15A).

c. Place a short, strong stick, or similar object that will not break, on the overhand knot and tie two additional overhand knots on top of the stick (Fig. 15B).

d. Twist the stick to tighten the tourniquet until bleeding stops (Fig. 15C).

e. Secure the stick in place with the loose ends of the tourniquet (Fig. 15D), a strip of cloth, or other improvised material (Fig. 15E).

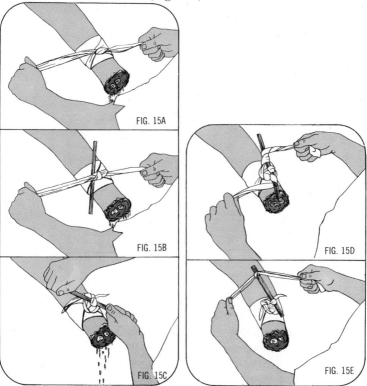

FIG. 15A

FIG. 15B

FIG. 15D

FIG. 15C

FIG. 15E

f. Make a written note of the location of the tourniquet and the time it was applied and attach the note to the victim's clothing.

g. Once the serious decision has been made to apply the tourniquet, *the tourniquet should not be loosened* except on the advice of a physician.

h. Treat the victim for shock, and give necessary first aid for other injuries.

Do not cover a tourniquet.

VI. PREVENTION OF CONTAMINATION AND INFECTION

Open wounds are subject to contamination and infection. The danger of infection can be prevented or lessened by taking the appropriate first aid measures, depending upon the severity of bleeding.

A. Safeguards

When a dressing has been applied to control bleeding, whether bleeding has been severe or not, safeguards must be taken.

1. Do not remove or disturb the cloth pad initially placed on the wound.

2. Do not attempt to cleanse the wound, since the victim requires medical care.

3. Attend to shock before and during transportation.

4. Immobilize the injured area.

5. When possible, adjust the victim's lying position so that the affected limb can be elevated.

B. Measures to take with wounds without severe bleeding

Wounds without severe bleeding that do not involve tissues deeper than the skin should be cleansed thoroughly. There will be some contamination, and it should be removed before the injury is dressed and bandaged, especially if medical attention is delayed. Removal of foreign materials in muscle or deep tissue should always be carried out by a physician.

1. To cleanse a wound, wash your hands thoroughly with soap and water. Use ordinary hand soap or mild detergent.

2. Wash in and around the victim's wound to remove bacteria and other foreign matter.

3. Rinse the wound thoroughly by flushing with clean water, preferably running tap water.

4. *Blot* the wound dry with a sterile gauze pad or a clean cloth.

5. Apply a dry sterile bandage or clean dressing and secure it firmly in place.

6. Caution the victim to see a physician promptly if evidence of infection appears (see page 33).

7. A physician may advise additional home remedies for the care of small wounds.

C. Removal of foreign objects

In small open wounds, wood splinters and glass fragments often remain in the skin tissues or in tissues just beneath the surface. Such objects, as a rule, only irritate the victim, but unless they are removed, they can cause infection.

1. Use tweezers, sterilized over a flame or in boiling water, to pull out any foreign matter from the surface tissue.

2. Objects imbedded just beneath the skin can be lifted out with the tip of a needle that has been sterilized in rubbing alcohol or in the heat of a flame.

3. Foreign objects, regardless of size, embedded deeper in the tissues should be left for removal by a physician.

4. The fishhook is probably one of the most common types of foreign objects that may penetrate the skin. Often, only the point of the hook enters, not penetrating deeply enough to allow the barb to become effective; in this case the hook can be removed easily by backing it out. If the fishhook goes deeper and the barb becomes embedded

(Fig. 16), the wisest course is to have a physician remove the hook. If medical aid is not available, remove the hook

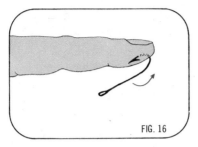

FIG. 16

by pushing it through (Fig. 17) until the barb protrudes. Using a cutting tool, cut the hook either at the barb or at

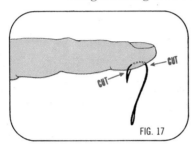

FIG. 17

the shank and remove it. Cleanse the wound thoroughly and cover it with an adhesive compress. A physician should be consulted as soon as possible because of the possibility of infection, especially tetanus.

5. Some penetrating foreign objects, such as sticks or pieces of metal, may protrude loosely from the body. Some penetrating objects, such as a stake in the ground or a spike of a fence, may be fixed and cause the victim to become impaled. Under no circumstances should the victim be pulled loose from a fixed object. Obtain help at once, preferably from ambulance or rescue personnel equipped to handle the problem. If the object is fixed or protrudes more than a few inches from the body, it should be left in place, be cut off at a distance from the skin, and be secured carefully to prevent movement that could cause further damage. If the victim must be transported, immobilize the protruding end with massive dressings around the protruding part, and then transport the victim to a hospital without delay and in the most comfortable manner possible.

D. Dressing the wound

A dressing is a cover placed over a wound to protect it from additional injury and contamination, and to assist in the control of bleeding. Bandaging a wound holds the dressing in place, assists in controlling the bleeding, offers support, and promotes restraint of movement. For detailed instruction on the application of dressings and bandages, see chapter 13.

E. Infection

The period of healing after an injury may be greatly lengthened by infection, which is the result of invasion and growth of bacteria within the tissues of the body. If bacteria get inside tissues of the body through breaks in the skin or mucous membranes, serious infection may develop within hours or days following an injury. The threat of tetanus infection, or lockjaw, must never be overlooked. Ask your physician whether or not a tetanus immunization or tetanus toxoid booster injection may be needed.

1. Symptoms

   a. Swelling of the affected part

   b. Redness of the affected part

   c. A sensation of heat

   d. Throbbing pain

   e. Tenderness

   f. Fever

   g. Evidence of pus, either collected beneath the skin or draining from the wound

   h. Swollen lymph glands, or "kernels," in the groin (leg infection), in the armpit (arm infection), or in the neck (infection in the head)

   i. Red streaks leading from the wound—an indication that the infection is spreading through the lymphatic circulation channels

2. Interim emergency care

   Prompt medical care is needed for an infected wound, but if any lengthy delay must occur before a physician can see the victim, the following temporary steps should be taken:

a. Keep victim lying down and quiet, and immobilize the entire infected area.

b. Elevate the affected body part, if possible.

c. Apply heat to the area with hot water bottles, or by placing warm, moist towels or cloths over the wound.

d. Do not delay efforts to get medical care for the victim. The above are interim measures only.

VII. Bites

Injuries produced by animal or human bites may cause punctures, lacerations, or even avulsions. Not only is care needed for open wounds but also consideration must be given to the danger of infection, especially rabies.

A. Human

Human bites that break the skin may become seriously infected, because the mouth is heavily contaminated with bacteria. Cleanse the wound thoroughly, cover it, and seek medical attention.

B. Animal

The bite of any animal, whether it is a wild animal or a pet, may result in an open wound. Dog and cat bites are common. Although a dog bite is likely to cause more extensive tissue damage than a cat bite, the cat bite may be more dangerous, because a wider variety of bacteria is usually present in the mouth of a cat. Many wild animals, especially bats, raccoons, and rats, transmit rabies. Rabies can be transmitted even when a rabid animal licks an existing open wound on a human or a nonrabid animal. Tetanus is an added danger in animal bites. Any animal bite carries a great risk of infection. There is no known cure for rabies, in human beings or in animals, once its final-stage symptoms develop. If the animal proves to be rabid, vaccine therapy must be given to build up body immunity in the victim in time to prevent the disease.

1. A bite of the face or neck should receive immediate medical attention.

2. Every effort must be made to restrain any suspected rabid animal so that it can be kept under observation to determine whether or not it develops the final stages of rabies. Find out from local health authorities how long a

live animal suspected of having rabies should be observed.

3. Do not kill the animal unless absolutely necessary. If the animal has to be killed, have the body examined for rabies. If killing is necessary, take precautions not to damage the animal's head.

4. If a suspected rabid animal cannot be caught or found and thus cannot be identified and observed, arrange for immediate medical care for any person it has bitten.

5. Injections are effective in preventing rabies in 95 percent of victims.

6. In the meantime, before the physician takes charge, thoroughly wash the wound with soap and water, flush the bitten area, and apply a dressing.

7. Make sure that the victim avoids movement of the affected part until he has been attended by a physician.

VIII. CLOSED WOUNDS

A. Characteristics

1. A closed wound may occur anywhere within the body.

2. There is no break in the skin.

3. Blood is not lost through the skin, but may flow through outer openings of body cavities.

4. Closed wounds are less likely to become infected than are open wounds, since they are subject to less contamination.

5. Many closed wounds are relatively small injuries involving soft tissue—the familiar black eye is an example. Other closed wounds, however, may involve extensive internal bleeding plus severe physical damage to tissues, organs, or systems.

B. Causes

1. Most closed wounds are caused by external forces, such as falls and motor vehicle accidents.

2. Sometimes closed wounds are caused if the victim of a closed fracture is mishandled or is moved before splints are properly applied to immobilize his injuries.

C. Signs and symptoms

1. General symptoms

Even if no outward signs of injury are obvious, internal injury is possible when any of the following general symptoms are present:

a. Cold, clammy, pale skin; very rapid but weak pulse; rapid breathing and dizziness.

b. Pain and tenderness in a part of the body in which injury is suspected, especially if deep pain continues and seems out of proportion to the injury symptoms.

c. Uncontrolled restlessness and excessive thirst.

d. Vomited or coughed-up blood, or blood in the urine or feces.

As a general rule, suspect a closed wound, with internal bleeding and possible rupture of a body organ, whenever a severe force exerted on the body produces severe shock or unconsciousness.

2. Specific symptoms

a. Pain

b. Tenderness

3. Signs

a. Swelling

b. Discoloration

c. Deformity of limbs, caused by fractures or dislocations.

D. Emergency care

1. Maintain an open airway; give artificial respiration if indicated.

2. Carefully examine the victim for fractures and other injuries to the head, neck, chest, abdomen, limbs, back, and spine.

3. If an internal injury is suspected, get medical care for the victim as soon as possible.

4. If a closed fracture is suspected, immobilize the affected

area before moving the victim.

5. If the victim must be moved, carefully transport him in a lying position; give special attention to preventing shock.

6. *Do not* give fluids by mouth to a victim suspected of having severe internal injury, no matter how much he complains of thirst.

7. When a relatively small closed wound occurs (such as a black eye), put cold applications on the injured area to prevent added tissue swelling and to slow down internal bleeding.

IX. PREVENTION OF WOUND-CAUSING ACCIDENTS

Almost any kind of accident may result in, or involve, a wound type of injury. Thus, it is very difficult to advise a person how to prevent accidents that cause wounds except on a broad, generalized basis. What follows concerns the more common wound-producing accidents that occur when a person is on the highway, at home, at work, or at play.

A. Categories

1. Highway accidents

Motor vehicle accidents are the leading cause of accidental death. In addition, each year, the number of persons who receive nonfatal injuries as a result of motor vehicle accidents is approximately 1 out of every 100 persons in the United States. Because of the great impact forces created by collisions of vehicles with each other, or with other moving or stationary objects, wounds resulting from such accidents are frequently severe in nature.

When a motor vehicle is in motion, the driver and passengers are also in an independent state of motion. If the vehicle should become involved in a collision, or suddenly change its direction or upright position, the driver and passengers continue to move forward essentially in a straight line and at a speed directly influenced by their weight and size plus the precrash speed of the vehicle. If the forward motion of a person's body is not restrained in some way, to prevent it from moving separately from the vehicle, the body will continue in motion as a separate missile until stopped by its own "secondary collision" with the metal, glass, or other material structure of the vehicle's interior. The impact obviously can produce wounds of varying type and severity.

It is impractical, if not impossible, to stop motor vehicle accidents by expecting people not to use such equipment and, thus, not to expose themselves to the hazards of riding in a moving vehicle. Preventive efforts, therefore, must be directed toward avoiding or controlling destructive forces that are created by a vehicle in motion. Four factors—engineering; regulatory laws; personal driving skill, knowledge, and judgment; and personal attitudes and practices about the highway rights of other drivers— are the main components of an effective approach toward avoiding or controlling destructive forces.

a. Engineering

The built-in safety features of motor vehicles and the roads on which the vehicles move depend primarily upon the caliber of engineering skill used to design, produce, and maintain them. Specific federal legislation was enacted in 1966 to authorize the issuance and implementation of "safety standards" for the design and manufacture of both vehicles and highways. However, to be effective, official actions need the positive support of the general public. The goal of safety could fail without such support.

Road surface and motor vehicle conditions are subject to change or breakdown. Be alert to posted or unexpected road hazards, and maintain your vehicle in good operating condition. Collapsible highway signs and deflecting guard rails have been substituted for previously used "immovable" objects. Vehicles have been built with collapsible steering columns, fly-away windshields, and devices for the driver and for passengers such as safety belts, shoulder harnesses, and head restraints.

Safety belts and body harnesses restrain independent forward momentum of a driver or passenger following vehicle impact. As a rule, put a motor vehicle in motion only after all occupants have strapped on protective devices.

b. Regulatory laws

The enactment and enforcement of regulatory laws
governing the operating of motor vehicles is a state and
local prerogative. However, the National Highway
Safety Act established criteria to be used by states in
strengthening their own requirements. Most state laws
are rather severe on violators, relative to speed and the
use of alcohol or drug inhibitors of driving skills. Periodic state or local inspections of vehicles, plus requirements for the issuance or reissuance of driving licenses,
are important aspects of highway safety.

c. Driving skill, knowledge, and judgment

Responsibility for control of a vehicle's speed and direction rests with the driver. The purpose of driver
education courses is to equip people with good driving
skills and enough real-life exposure to normal traffic
conditions to help individual drivers learn the basics of
driving judgment and the application of judgment to
the many unexpected emergencies that can develop
suddenly while driving.

d. Personal attitudes, practices, and behavior

Vehicle safety devices and highway signs become useless unless they are used. Therefore, use them; they are
for your safety.

Traffic laws are enacted not to penalize people but to
protect oneself and others from the potentially destructive forces of a motor vehicle in motion. Therefore,
know and obey traffic laws; support and cooperate
with law enforcement efforts; and encourage legislation
that will improve highway safety. Excessive speed by
younger drivers and right-of-way violations in the case
of older drivers are the most frequent improper driving
practices that lead to motor vehicle accidents. It is
apparent that many highway accidents could be prevented by the routine use of common courtesy toward
other drivers.

For your own safety and that of others, take specific

actions that could significantly prevent or reduce motor
vehicle accidents:

- Use seat and shoulder belts at all times.
- Use safe driving and walking practices.
- Drive defensively.
- Keep your vehicle in proper working condition by
  having the brakes, lights, windshield wipers, tires,
  and steering mechanism checked regularly.
- Avoid drugs that cause drowsiness.
- Avoid alcohol; do not drive when you drink.
- Take frequent breaks on long trips and stop when
  you are tired or sleepy.
- Obey traffic regulations.
- Always signal your intention to turn or stop.

2. Home and work accidents

Home accidents rank second to motor vehicle accidents as
a leading cause of accidental death. More nonfatal injuries
occur in the home each year than in any other environment in which a person works, plays, or moves about.
Many such injuries are wounds and are received within
the home environment, usually as the result of the improper use or handling of physical objects.

Occupational accidents cause fewer deaths and permanent disabilities than do motor vehicle or home accidents.
However, more than half of the injuries suffered by workers occur off, not on, the job. Wounds received in the
work environment result frequently from mishandling of
physical objects, falls, being struck by moving or falling
objects, and machinery.

Many conditions and activities that produce wounds at
home are also present in the work environment. Tools,
implements, appliances, and machinery are used in both
places.

Accessibility to sharp, jagged, or pointed objects creates
similar housekeeping, storage, and safeguarding requirements. The necessity for learning, guidance, supervision,
and behavioral control exists at home as well as on the job.
Knowledge, skill, experience, and judgment factors affect
the accident potential in both environments.

A great variety of physical objects that are potentially destructive to body tissue can be found in any home or place of employment. In both environments people frequently move about within a relatively confined space. Conditions and activities that can produce forceful impact between the body and some physical object are, therefore, ever present. Preventive efforts must be directed toward the elimination, control, and avoidance of the source, direction, and amount of tissue-destructive forces.

Appliances and machinery can create tissue-destructive forces of varying intensity. Although they contain built-in safeguards, instructions for their safe and efficient operation is usually given in printed warnings and instructions. Handle such items according to the manufacturer's directions, and use recommended protective devices.

Sharp, jagged, or pointed objects require relatively little penetrating force to break skin tissue. When using such an object, direct its penetrating force away from the body or body parts. Keep such objects safely secured from unsuspecting hands and feet. When they are carried by hand from one place to another, make certain that conditions or activities that may cause a person to fall on the subject are eliminated. Protect children who lack knowledge and handling skill by keeping such objects out of sight or reach.

Tools and implements are, in most cases, designed to perform specific tasks. The amount of their cutting, turning, prying, drilling, or driving force potential is limited by design features. Use tools and implements only for their intended purposes.

Explosive forces generally produce wounds of considerable depth and destruction. Use of firearms and explosives should be carefully controlled. Safe and proper handling of explosive devices or materials requires specialized training and careful supervision. Unsupervised use should be restricted to persons highly skilled and having knowledge of the control of the destructive capability of explosive forces. Make every possible effort to secure or safeguard the source of any explosive force from unauthorized or unsuspecting hands.

Concern for occupational safety and health led to the

Williams-Steiger Occupational Safety and Health Act of 1970, which authorizes the development and enforcement of standards to assure safe and healthful working conditions for employees. In general, the standards are rules for the avoidance of hazards that have been proved by research and experience to be harmful to personal safety and health. The act requires all employers and employees to become familiar with its standards and to abide by those standards that apply to them. The responsibility for promulgating and enforcing job safety and health standards has been assigned to the Secretary of Labor.

3. Leisure-time accidents

Leisure-time play activities provide people with an opportunity to relieve tensions and anxiety. Off-duty and away-from-home pursuits place people in a wide variety of accident-producing conditions and activities. Such conditions and activities may be spontaneous or planned, informal or structured, uninhibited or supervised. They take place in environments both natural and unnatural to man. Accident-producing actions may involve running, climbing, striking, throwing, jumping, soaring, building, riding, swimming, or similar activities in which people and physical objects are in motion.

Most games, sports, and play activities either create or take place within a situation where forces destructive of tissue and bone are present. Types and severities of injuries are equally varied, but wounds commonly result. Unfortunately, the effort required to prevent accidents when people are at play often is ignored in the quest for pleasure and personal satisfaction. But accident prevention efforts must be made to develop proper regard for safety without sacrifice of the personal satisfaction and pleasure that people seek from recreational activities.

Most wounds that occur in a play environment result from falling, running into an object, or being struck by a thrown or swung object. Elimination, control, or avoidance of such impact forces involves awareness of hazards, degree of performance skill, structural and mechanical factors, regard for rules and regulations, guidance and supervision, physical and mental capabilities, environmental conditions, and the use of protective equipment or devices.

Climbing is a natural form of spontaneous play among children. It becomes an unsafe activity whenever dangers such as poor footing and gripping, or structural weakness, go unrecognized or are ignored. Help children to recognize and understand such hazards. Give them direction and guidance that may be necessary to prevent a fall, particularly when constant supervision is impractical.

Informal play frequently exposes young children to unfamiliar conditions and dangerous activities. While exploring strange surroundings and experimenting with new objects, children often fail to look beyond the pleasure and personal satisfaction of the moment. Provide enough supervision of informal play to protect children against hazards they may fail to recognize.

Impact on the body is often expected in formal games or sports that find people or physical objects in motion, but rules and regulations help to protect participants from excessive impact forces. Instruction promotes, and supervision permits, control of dangerous forces. Ability to avoid tissue-destructive force is enhanced by good performance skill, use of recommended protective devices, and provision of a suitable play environment. A proper regard for safety increases the enjoyment of games and sports.

Adults also are predisposed to tissue-destructive forces in their active leisure-time pursuits. Recreational opportunities and interests continue to expand. More and more persons are performing their own home care and repair activities. Know your skill and physical limitations. Handle and use equipment with due respect for its limitations, and with proper concern for self-protection and the protection of others.

B. Preventive measures

The following specific actions may significantly prevent or reduce wound-causing accidents:

- Use sharp objects only for their intended purpose, handle them with care, and keep them out of the reach of children.
- Do not allow children to run with wooden sticks or with articles that may break if the children fall (for example, bottles, glasses, or plastic toys).

- Mark or identify large picture walk-through doors so that unsuspecting individuals will see them and not walk into them.
- Evaluate as sources of injury all household appliances and equipment for work or play, including power tools, lawn-mowers, and all electrical equipment.
- Follow the manufacturer's instructions carefully when using equipment.
- Unplug electric cords when equipment is not in use.
- Instruct children not to play with or around television sets, electrical devices in the kitchen and bathroom, fans, power tools, household cleaning equipment, sewing machines, lawn tools, and other dangerous objects.
- Be a good housekeeper and check the home frequently for objects that may cause lacerations or puncture wounds.
- Sweep up broken glass promptly. Discard cracked china and glassware. Use nonbreakable dishes and containers for all children and around tile and cement surfaces.
- Remove nails from boards.
- Keep yards, garages, storage rooms, basements, and play areas free of trash and bottles.
- Take special precautions with firearms and ammunition and observe safety rules.
- Keep guns and ammunition in separate places, each protected by lock and key.
- Do not allow children to play with any guns, including pellet and BB guns.
- *Assume* that all guns, as you handle them, are loaded but *never* load a gun until you are ready to shoot it. Do not misuse blank cartridges; they can cause serious injury and even death.
- Do not allow children to play with fireworks. Avoid the temptation to show off with fireworks in front of them.

3

SPECIFIC INJURIES

I. EYE INJURIES

Foreign objects are often blown or rubbed into the eyes. Such objects are harmful not only because of the irritating effect but also because of the danger of their scratching the surface or becoming embedded in the eye.

A. Symptoms

    1. Redness of eyes

    2. Burning sensation

    3. Pain

    4. Headache

    5. Overproduction of tears

B. Precautions

    1. Keep the victim from rubbing his eye.

    2. Wash your hands thoroughly before examining the victim's eye.

    3. Do not attempt to remove a foreign object by inserting a match, toothpick, or any other instrument.

    4. Refer the victim to a physician if something is embedded in the eye, or if something is thought to be embedded but cannot be located.

C. Removal of a foreign body from the surface of the eyeball or from the inner surface of the eyelid

1. Pull down the lower lid to determine whether or not the object lies on the inner surface.

2. If the object lies on the inner surface, lift it gently with the corner of a clean handkerchief or paper tissue. Never use dry cotton around the eye.

3. If the object has not been located, it may be lodged beneath the upper lid.

     a. While the victim looks down, grasp the lashes of the upper lid gently.

     b. Pull the upper lid forward and down over the lower lid. Tears may dislodge the foreign object.

     c. If the foreign object has not been dislodged, depress the victim's upper lid with a matchstick (Fig. 18A) or similar object placed horizontally on the top of the cartilage and evert the lid, by pulling upward on the lashes against the matchstick (Fig. 18B). Lift off the foreign

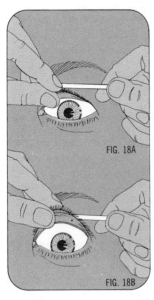

FIG. 18A

FIG. 18B

     object with the corner of a clean handkerchief and replace the lid by pulling downward gently on the lashes.

     d. Flush the eye with water.

e. If the object is still not removed and is suspected to be embedded, apply a dry, protective dressing and consult a physician.

D. Injuries

1. Injury of the eyelid

First aid in injury of the eyelid as follows:

a. Stop hemorrhage by gently applying direct pressure.

b. Cleanse the wound and apply a sterile or clean dressing, which can be taped in place or held snugly by a bandage that encircles the head. Seek medical care without delay.

c. Bruises above and below the eye, involving rupture of small blood vessels, should be treated by immediate cold applications to lessen bleeding and swelling.

2. Blunt injury or contusion

a. A contusion occurs from a direct blow, as from a fist, a vehicle accident, or an explosion. The most common result is a black eye.

b. In serious cases, the structure of the eye may be torn or ruptured.

c. Secondary damage may be produced by the effects of hemorrhage, and later by infection.

d. Vision may be lost.

e. Bleeding may recur after several days.

f. Any person experiencing a blunt injury of the eye should be seen by a physician, preferably an eye specialist, as soon as possible.

g. A dry sterile or clean dressing should be applied, and the victim should be transported lying flat.

3. Penetrating injuries of the eye

Penetrating injuries of the eye are extremely serious and can result in blindness. First aid is as follows:

a. Make no attempt to remove the object or to wash the eye.

b. Cover both eyes loosely with a sterile or clean dressing, secured with tape or a bandage that encircles the victim's head but loose enough to avoid pressure on the eyes. Coverage of *both* eyes is necessary to eliminate movement of the affected eye.

c. Keep the victim quiet, preferably on his back.

d. Transport the victim by stretcher.

e. Telephone ahead to an eye specialist, or take the victim to the nearest appropriate hospital emergency room. The sooner he receives medical care, the greater the chances of saving his sight.

II. HEAD INJURIES

A. Scalp injuries

1. Characteristics

Wounds of the scalp, even if small, tend to bleed profusely. A severe wound may be concealed by thick hair and therefore be overlooked. Deep scalp wounds may be complicated by fragments from skull fractures, or they may contain hair, glass, or other foreign matter.

2. First aid

a. Do not attempt to cleanse scalp wounds of contaminants; to do so may cause serious bleeding and, if the skull is fractured, can lead to contamination of the brain.

b. Control bleeding by raising the victim's head and shoulders, if possible; but do not bend the neck, since a fracture may be present.

c. Place a sterile dressing snugly on the wound. Excessive pressure should not be used, however, because the bone may be fractured.

d. When bleeding is under control, apply a bandage to hold the dressing in place and to provide continuing pressure.

B. Brain injuries

Brain injury may be a factor not only in wounds of the scalp and open or closed fractures of the skull but also in the case of an illness such as a stroke or a tumor.

1. Symptoms

    a. Clear or blood-tinged cerebrospinal fluid draining from the nose or ears following a skull fracture

    b. Temporary loss of consciousness (If a person with a head injury loses consciousness later, his condition is probably serious because of progressive swelling of the brain or a hemorrhage within the skull.)

    c. Other manifestations of brain injury

        (1) Partial or complete paralysis of muscles of the extremities of the opposite side, and the muscles of the face on the same side as the side of the brain injury

        (2) Disturbance of speech

        (3) Convulsions, general or local, indicated by persistent twitching of muscles

        (4) Bleeding from the nose, ear canal, or mouth, which reflects possible head injury with a fracture

        (5) A pale or flushed face

        (6) Pulse, although slow and full initially, becoming fast and weak

        (7) Headache, sometimes associated with dizziness

        (8) Vomiting

        (9) Pupils of the eyes unequal in size

        (10) Loss of bowel and bladder control

2. <u>First aid</u> for suspected brain injury

    a. Obtain medical assistance as quickly as possible. Call for an ambulance equipped with oxygen.

    b. Keep the victim lying down. Treat for shock and if there is no evidence of neck injury and the victim is unconscious, place a small pillow or a pillow substitute (for example, a rolled-up blanket or overcoat) under his shoulders and head. *Do not* place the pillow only under the victim's head, because doing so might result in head flexion with consequent airway obstruction. Turn his head toward the side so that secretions may drool from the corner of his mouth. Never position the victim so that his head is lower than the rest of his body. Remove the pillow if artificial respiration is to be used.

   c. Give particular attention to ensuring an open airway. Administer artificial respiration when necessary.

   d. Control hemorrhage.

   e. *Do not* give the victim fluids by mouth.

   f. If a scalp wound is present, apply a large dressing over the injury and bandage it in place with a full head bandage.

   g. Record the extent and duration of unconsciousness.

C. Face and jaw injuries

  1. Causes

Wounds and fractures of the face and of the upper or lower jaw often occur in victims of automobile accidents or other types of violent injury.

  2. First aid

The principal immediate problems are obstruction of the air passage by blood, saliva, and other secretions; and swelling and severe hemorrhage.

   a. Have someone call for an ambulance or medical assistance as quickly as possible.

   b. Continuously maintain an open airway. Remove any dentures, broken teeth, or other foreign matter.

   c. Provide continuous support of the victim's head and jaw to prevent airway obstruction by the tongue.

   d. If the victim is conscious and neck injury is not suspected, prop him up so that he is leaning forward to let secretions drain out spontaneously or when he coughs. If the facial injuries are extensive, the victim should be assumed to have a cervical spine fracture until X rays prove otherwise.

e. If the victim is unconscious, elevate his head and shoulders slightly (unless neck fracture is suspected) and turn his head to the side to allow blood and saliva to drain out, or place him on his side or abdomen for drainage.

f. Apply artificial respiration if necessary.

NOTE. Jaw fractures and injuries that cause bleeding from the mouth or nose create special problems if artificial respiration is given. Proper positioning and the gentle removal of foreign material or of blood clots may help to ensure an open airway, but the injuries may be such that it is difficult or impossible to administer mouth-to-mouth or mouth-to-nose artificial respiration.

Under extremely rare conditions, the first-aider may have to resort to an alternate manual method of artificial respiration (see page 81).

g. Treat for shock.

h. Apply protective dressings as necessary.

D. Ear injuries

1. Cuts and lacerations

Cuts and lacerations of the ear occur frequently. Any torn and detached part of the ear should be saved and should accompany the victim to a medical facility. First aid is as follows:

a. Apply a dressing with light, even pressure.

b. Raise the victim's head.

2. Perforation

a. Causes

Perforation (rupture) of the eardrum may result from a blast, a blow on the head, diving, a sudden change in atmospheric pressure, or a disease of the middle ear.

b. First aid

(1) Place a small pledget of gauze or cotton loosely in the outer ear canal for protection.

(2) Obtain medical care.

(3) Do not allow the victim to hit himself on the side of his head in an effort to restore hearing.

(4) Do not insert instruments or any kind of liquid into the ear canal.

3. Perforation of the eardrum associated with skull fracture

   a. Precaution

   Perforation of eardrum associated with skull fracture requires special attention.

   b. First aid

   (1) Do not clean the ear.

   (2) Do not stop the flow of cerebrospinal fluid from the ear.

   (3) Turn the victim onto his injured side (unless there is some reason not to do so), with his head and shoulders propped up on a small pillow to allow fluid to drain away.

E. Nose injuries and nosebleeds

1. Characteristics and causes

   Injury to the soft tissue of the nose may or may not include fractures. Nosebleeds can result from injury or disease (such as high blood pressure, which can cause profuse, prolonged, and dangerous bleeding). Nosebleed may also occur after a cold, a period of strenuous activity, or exposure to high altitudes. Nosebleeds are generally more annoying than serious. Walking, talking, laughing, blowing the nose, or otherwise disturbing clots may cause increase or resumption of bleeding.

2. First aid

   a. Keep the victim quiet.

   b. Place the victim in a sitting position, leaning forward if possible; if that is not possible, place him in a reclining position with the head and shoulders raised.

   c. Apply pressure directly at the site of bleeding by pressing the bleeding nostril toward the midline.

   d. Apply cold compresses to the victim's nose and face.

   e. If bleeding cannot be controlled by the preceding measures, insert a small, clean pad of gauze (not absorbent cotton) into one or both nostrils and apply pressure externally with your thumb and index finger. A free end of the pad must extend outside the nostril so that the pad can be removed later.

   f. If bleeding continues, obtain medical assistance.

   g. Do not use first aid measures against the injury itself except, perhaps, a dressing.

   h. Make sure that nasal bone fractures, like all other fractures, have medical attention.

III. NECK INJURIES

A. Blockage of the airway

Blunt force exerted on the face, mouth, or jaw may produce so much tissue damage that body fluids draining into the air passages block the airway. The airway may also be blocked as a result of a hard blow on the front of the neck, especially if the larynx area is affected and throat tissues are bruised so badly that extensive swelling results. In such cases, if necessary, do the following:

1. Apply mouth-to-mouth or mouth-to-nose artificial respiration.

2. Obtain immediate medical assistance, in case of emergency tracheostomy (an opening into the trachea) is needed.

B. Lacerations or puncture wounds

Lacerations or puncture wounds of the neck may involve the jugular veins, which are on the sides of the neck just beneath the skin, or the deeper major arteries and veins. Bleeding from neck wounds is dangerous and difficult to control. Control bleeding by the following measures:

1. Exert direct pressure over the wound.

2. Keep the victim's head and shoulders raised and his airway open.

3. Do not remove pressure until the victim is seen by a physician.

4. Seek medical attention without delay.

5. If bleeding is not a problem, cover wound with a dressing held in place with tape.

6. Never apply a circular bandage around the neck.

IV. WOUNDS OF THE CHEST

A. Sucking wound of the chest

1. Description and precautions

A sucking wound of the chest is a deep, open wound of the chest wall through which air can flow in and out with breathing (Fig. 19). If the wounding object or instrument

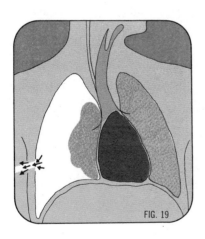

FIG. 19

is still in place, leave it undisturbed; removing it may result in fatal bleeding. The victim should be taken as quickly as possible to the nearest hospital. The hospital staff should be alerted in advance, if possible, and be told the nature of the emergency.

2. <u>First aid</u>

    a. To prevent air from entering the cavity, cover the open wound by placing a large pad over the opening. The pad may be made from sterile gauze, a cloth as clean as possible, plastic, or metal foil. The pad should form an airtight seal and should be held in place with tape, a belt, or a bandage. Be careful, however, not to apply the binding so tightly that breathing is restricted.

    b. If necessary, the palm of the hand may be applied until a suitable bandage can be obtained.

    c. Maintain an open airway and give artificial respiration if required.

    d. Transport the victim with his injured side down.

B. Penetrating wounds of the heart or the large blood vessel of the chest

1. Precautions

If the victim has been injured by an object or instrument that penetrates the body and remains there, the penetrating object should be left undisturbed and immobilized in place with dressings and tape if possible.

2. <u>First aid</u>

    a. Elevate the victim's head.

    b. Give artificial respiration if necessary.

    c. Take the victim as quickly as possible to the nearest hospital. The staff should be alerted in advance and told of the nature of the emergency.

C. Compression of lung tissue

1. Causes and precautions

A lung may be compressed by blood or other fluids, or by air that has escaped into the chest cavity from air passages through a tear in the surface of the lung. This is an emergency that requires *immediate* medical attention, but until medical attention is available, any person with difficulty in breathing should have first aid, as described below.

2. First aid

   a. Position the victim for mouth-to-mouth artificial respiration. Maintain an open airway.

   b. Give artificial respiration if necessary.

   c. Seek medical help as quickly as possible.

D. Crushing injuries of the chest

   1. Causes and characteristics

   Crushing injuries of the chest are commonly found in victims of vehicle accidents, when the driver comes in contact with the steering wheel, for example. Crushing injuries of the chest with multiple rib fractures tend to restrict breathing because of extreme pain, thus reducing the volume of air reaching the lungs.

   2. First aid

   First Aid measures include placing the victim in a comfortable position. If fractures are on one side, place the victim on the injured side, if possible. If a bandage is required for an open wound, apply it carefully, so as not to interfere with breathing. Elevation of the victim's head and shoulders may reduce his difficulty in breathing.

V. ABDOMINAL INJURIES

A. Precaution

Wounds of the abdomen are particularly dangerous because of the risk of damage to internal organs.

B. First aid

   1. Wounds deep in the abdomen

      a. Place the victim at rest on his back (supine position) with a pillow under the knees to help relax the abdominal muscles.

      b. Control bleeding.

      c. Give first aid for shock.

  2. Open wounds of the abdomen

      a. Do not try to replace protruding intestines or abdominal organs but cover them with a sterile dressing, a clean towel, plastic, or metal foil. Dampen the dressing if there is delay in obtaining medical assistance; use sterile water or cool, boiled water, if available.

      b. Hold the dressing in place with a firm bandage, but do not apply the bandage so tightly as to cause constriction.

      c. Do not give fluids or solid food, because surgery will be necessary.

      d. If breathing is difficult, keep the victim's head and shoulders elevated with a pillow or a folded coat.

      e. Summon medical attention as rapidly as possible and take extreme care to gently transport the victim.

VI. BACK INJURIES

In any accident involving the back, injury to the spinal cord should be considered. Careful handling of the victim is extremely important. Do not bend the back during transportation. If the victim requires artificial respiration, it should begin in the position in which he is lying. A person who has been injured in the water should not have his head bent forward, nor should he be placed in a jackknife position. The victim should be floated to shore carefully and should be taken from the water only when a rigid support is available. Preferably, the victim should not be moved until an ambulance arrives with a special stretcher and trained personnel.

VII. INJURIES TO THE GENITAL ORGANS

  A. Causes and characteristics

Injuries to the genital organs may result from kicks, blows, straddle accidents, accidents involving machinery, and occasionally blows from sharp instruments. Such injuries are accompanied by great pain, marked swelling, and considerable bleeding.

B. First aid

1. Save any torn tissue for possible skin grafting.

2. Control bleeding by direct pressure with the hand on a pad of cloth.

3. Give first aid for shock, if appropriate.

4. Provide protective and supportive dressings for open wounds.

5. Apply cold packs, if available.

6. Provide bed rest.

VIII. INJURIES TO LEGS AND FEET

A. Precautions and characteristics

Serious wounds of the legs and feet are obviously incapacitating, but the importance of small wounds of the lower legs and feet is frequently overlooked. In older persons, small wounds may take a long time to heal because of poor circulation.

B. First aid

Such injuries should receive medical attention, but if medical treatment is delayed—

1. Cover wounds of the legs and feet and wrap them with supportive—not constrictive—bandages if available.

2. Keep an injured limb elevated with pillows or a rolled-up coat.

3. Do not allow the victim with a leg or foot wound to walk.

4. Remove shoes and hose and examine color of the toes from time to time. If toes become blue or swollen, loosen the bandages but do not remove dressings.

IX. HAND INJURIES—FIRST AID

A. The most important first aid for a hand injury is elevation above the level of the heart, in order to reduce further swelling of tissues caused by gravity. (Only after snakebite and stings should the hand be kept hanging down after injury.)

B. If the wound is at all serious, do not try to cleanse it.

C. Apply pressure over a sterile or clean pad to control bleeding; place a role of bandage or cloth, fluffed-up gauze squares, or other material into the palm of the victim's hand and curve his fingers around it.

D. Separate the fingers by gauze or cloth dressing material and cover the entire hand with a sterile towel, a clean cloth, or an unused plastic bag.

E. Elevate the victim's hand in a sling or on pillows during transportation to receive medical care.

X. BLISTERS—FIRST AID

A. Blisters caused by friction from shoes or boots appear on the heels, toes, and tops of feet. If *all* pressure can be relieved until the fluid is absorbed, blisters are best left unbroken. Otherwise, wash the entire area with soap and water and make a small puncture hole at the base of the blister with a needle that has been sterilized in a match flame or by soaking in rubbing alcohol.

B. Apply a sterile dressing and protect the area from further irritation.

C. If the blister has already broken, treat it as an open wound. Watch for signs of infection.

D. Self-care for blisters *should not be attempted* when the blister fluid lies deep in the palm of the hand or sole of the foot.

4

SHOCK

I. DEFINITION

Shock is a condition resulting from a depressed state of many vital body functions, a depression that could threaten life even though the victim's injuries would not otherwise be fatal.

Injury-related shock, commonly referred to as traumatic shock, is decidedly different from electrical shock, insulin shock, and other special forms of shock.

II. CAUSES

A. Shock may be caused by severe injuries of all types; hemorrhage, or loss of body fluids other than blood (as in prolonged vomiting, dysentery, or burns); infection; heart attack or stroke; or poisoning by chemicals, gases, alcohol, or drugs. Shock also results from lack of oxygen, caused by obstruction of air passages or injury to the respiratory system.

B. The degree of shock is increased by abnormal changes in body temperature and by poor resistance of the victim to stress.

C. Shock is aggravated by pain, by rough handling, and by delay in treatment.

III. SIGNS AND SYMPTOMS

A. Early stages

In the early stages of shock, the body compensates for a

decreased blood flow to the tissues by constricting the blood vessels in the skin, soft tissues, and skeletal muscles. The following signs may develop as a result:

1. The skin is pale (or bluish) and cold to the touch. In the care of victims with dark skin, it may be necessary to rely primarily on the color of the mucous membranes on the inside of the mouth or under the eyelids, or of the nail beds.

2. The skin may be moist and clammy if perspiration has occurred.

3. The victim is weak.

4. The pulse is usually quite rapid (over 100) and often too faint to be felt at the wrist (Fig. 20A) but perceptible in the carotid artery at the side of the neck (Fig. 20B) or in the femoral artery at the groin (see Fig. 12, page 26).

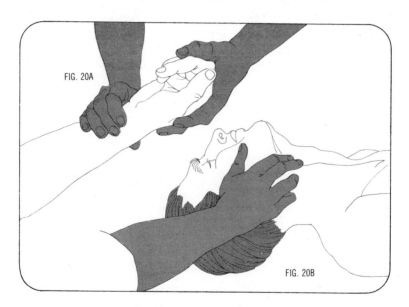

FIG. 20A

FIG. 20B

5. The rate of breathing is usually increased; it may be shallow, possibly deep, and irregular.

6. If there has been injury to the chest or abdomen, breathing will almost certainly be shallow, because of the pain involved in breathing deeply.

7. A victim in shock from hemorrhage may be restless and anxious (early signs of oxygen lack), thrashing about, and complaining of severe thirst.

8. The victim may vomit or retch from nausea.

B. Late stages

If the victim's condition deteriorates, the following additional signs may be noted:

1. The victim becomes apathetic and relatively unresponsive.

2. The victim's eyes are sunken, with a vacant expression, and his pupils may be widely dilated (Fig. 21).

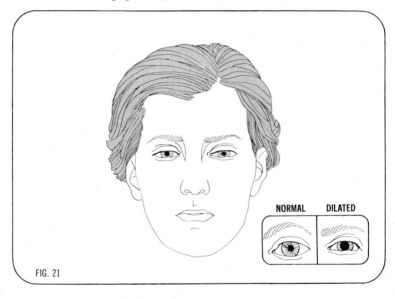

FIG. 21

3. Some of the blood vessels in the skin may be congested, producing a mottled appearance, which indicates the victim's blood pressure has fallen to a very low level.

4. If untreated, the victim eventually loses consciousness, his body temperature falls, and he may die.

IV. TREATMENT OBJECTIVES

A. To improve circulation of the blood

B. To ensure an adequate supply of oxygen

C. To maintain normal body temperature

V. FIRST AID

Give urgently necessary first aid immediately to eliminate the causes of shock, such as stoppage of breathing, hemorrhaging, or severe pain.

A. Steps for preventing shock and for giving first aid

    1. Keep the victim lying down.

    2. Cover him *only* enough to keep him from losing body heat.

    3. Get medical help as soon as possible.

B. Body position

    1. The position for a victim must be based on his injuries. Generally, the most satisfactory position for the injured person will be lying down to improve the circulation of blood.

    2. If injuries of the neck or lower spine are suspected, *do not* move the victim until he is properly prepared for transportation, unless it is necessary to protect him from further injury or to provide urgent first aid care.

    3. A victim with severe wounds of the lower part of the face and jaw, or who is unconscious, should be placed on his side to allow drainage of fluids and to avoid blockage of the airway by vomitus and blood (Fig. 22). Extreme care must be taken to ensure an open airway and to prevent

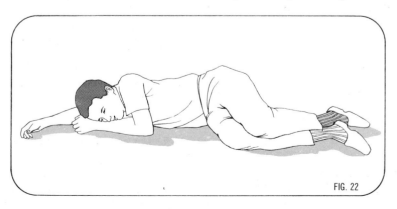

FIG. 22

asphyxia. When there is no danger of aspiration of fluids, a victim who is having difficulty breathing may be placed on his back with his head and shoulders raised (Fig. 23).

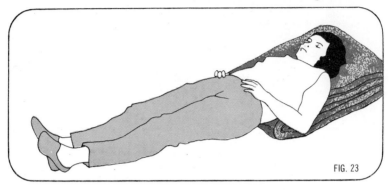

FIG. 23

4. A person with a head injury may be kept flat or propped up, but his head must not be lower than the rest of his body.

5. If in doubt concerning the proper position of the victim based on injuries sustained, keep him lying flat.

6. Victims in shock may improve if the feet (or foot of the stretcher) are raised from 8 to 12 inches (Fig. 24). If the

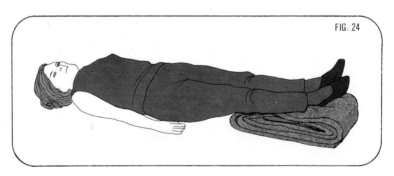

FIG. 24

victim has increased difficulty in breathing or experiences additional pain after his feet are raised, lower the feet again.

C. Regulating body temperature

Keep the victim warm enough to avoid or overcome chilling. If the victim is exposed to cold or dampness, blankets or additional clothing should be placed over and under him to

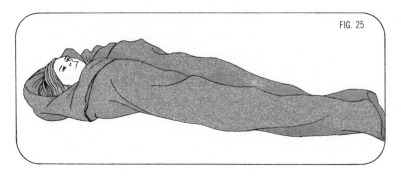

FIG. 25

prevent chilling (Fig. 25). No attempt should be made to add extra heat, because raising the surface temperature of the body is harmful.

D. Administering fluids

1. Giving fluids by mouth has value in shock, but fluids should only be given when medical help is not available within a reasonable time. Fluids should not be given, however, when victims are unconscious, are vomiting or are likely to vomit, or are having convulsions, since victims in such states may aspirate fluids into the lungs.

2. Do not give fluids when a victim is likely to require surgery or general anesthetic, or when he appears to have a brain or abdominal injury.

3. Fluids may be given by mouth only if medical care is delayed for an hour or more and no contraindications exist. Water that is neither hot nor cold—preferably a salt-soda solution (containing 1 level teaspoonful of salt and 1/2 level teaspoonful of baking soda to each quart of water) should be given as follows:

   a. An adult victim should be given about 4 ounces (1/2 glass) every 15 minutes.

   b. Approximately 2 ounces should be given to children aged from 1 to 12, and 1 ounce to infants of 1 year or less.

   c. Discontinue fluids if the victim becomes nauseated or vomits.

5

RESPIRATORY EMERGENCIES AND ARTIFICIAL RESPIRATION

I. DEFINITIONS

  A. Respiratory emergency

    A respiratory emergency is one in which normal breathing stops or in which breathing is so reduced that oxygen intake is insufficient to support life.

  B. Artificial respiration

    Artificial respiration is a procedure for causing air to flow into and out of a person's lungs when his natural breathing is inadequate or ceases.

II. CAUSES OF RESPIRATORY FAILURE

  A. Anatomic obstruction

    1. Obstruction by tongue

      The most common cause of respiratory emergency is interference with breathing caused by the tongue's dropping back and obstructing the throat.

    2. Other causes of obstruction that constrict the air passages

      a. Acute asthma

      b. Croup

      c. Diphtheria

      d. Spasm of the larynx

e. Swelling after burns of the face

f. Swallowing of corrosive poisons

g. Direct injury caused by a blow

B. Mechanical obstruction

1. Partial or complete blockage of the air passage by a solid foreign object lodged in the pharynx or in any part of the airway

Sudden death may occur from obstruction of the air passages directly or by pressure of a foreign body within the esophagus, which lies behind the trachea. In some instances of choking on food, a diagnosis of heart attack has been made on the basis of the victim's sudden collapse with marked chest pain, difficulty in breathing, and bluish discoloration of the face. A true life-threatening emergency exists when a person is choking and having difficulty in breathing. If he is unable to speak, it is a sure indication that the larynx is obstructed.

2. Accumulation of fluids in the back of the throat (mucus, blood, or saliva, for example)

3. Inhalation of vomitus

C. Air depleted of oxygen or containing toxic gases

1. Causes of asphyxia

Asphyxia may occur from breathing air that does not contain sufficient oxygen, or air containing carbon monoxide or other toxic gas. Natural, slow oxidation processes sometimes remove oxygen from the air in such places as wells, cisterns, sewers, mines, and silos.

If air does not contain oxygen, it will not support life, whether toxic gases are present or not. Plastic bags and other materials that may cause asphyxia when placed over the nose and mouth should be kept out of the reach of small children. Refrigerators and freezers, frequently implicated in accidents to children, should never be abandoned unless the doors have been removed.

2. Explosion hazard

In addition to the dangers of asphyxia from carbon monoxide, or from displacement of oxygen by natural oxidation processes or by other gases, there is often an explosion hazard. Combustible gases that accumulate in confined spaces—such as mines, cisterns, and sewers, or in rooms where natural or manufactured gas is free in the air—are explosive in certain concentrations. The explosion may result if a flame is introduced, if static electricity is discharged, or if an electric switch, doorbell, telephone, or other device is used.

3. Additional causes of respiratory failure

   a. Electrocution

   b. Drowning

   c. Circulatory collapse (shock)

   d. Heart disease

   e. External strangulation, as in hanging

   f. Compression of the chest (caused, for example, by a mine cave-in)

   g. Disease or injury to the lungs (Inadequate ventilation may be caused by injuries that collapse or compress lung tissue, injuries that permit air to enter through a sucking wound of the chest wall, accumulation of blood in the chest cavity from hemorrhage, or by inflammatory diseases of the lung such as pneumonia.)

   h. Poisoning by respiration-depressing drugs, such as morphine, opium, codeine, barbiturates, and alcohol

III. THE BREATHING PROCESS

Contraction of chest muscles and diaphragm causes enlargement of the chest cavity. (The diaphragm is a muscular partition forming the floor of the chest cavity, separating the chest cavity from the abdomen.)

A. Inhalation phase

   1. The muscles of the chest lift the ribs, expanding the chest.

2. The diaphragm, which is dome-shaped, contracts and descends toward the abdomen (Fig. 26).

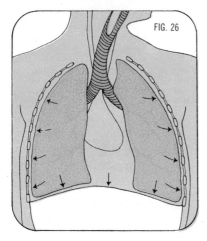

FIG. 26

In this way the chest cavity is increased in size, and atmospheric air flows in.

B. Exhalation phase

1. The muscles relax, allowing the ribs and diaphragm to resume their former positions.

2. The chest cavity becomes smaller, and air flows outward (Fig. 27)

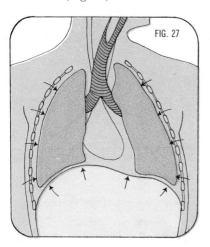

FIG. 27

C. Rate of breathing

   1. In adults, the rate of breathing, at rest, is about from 12 to 18 times per minute.

   2. The rate of breathing is somewhat faster in children and varies greatly with exercise, excitement, and disease.

   3. Approximately 1 pint of air is inhaled with each breath by resting adults, but not all of this air actually enters the lung tissue.

For artificial respiration to be effective, the volume of air that enters must exceed the amount that is already in the air passages and that is needed for normal respiration. Hence, air should be forced into the victim.

D. Need for oxygen

The body does not store oxygen but needs a continuous, fresh supply to carry on the life processes.

Oxygen must be available to all body cells and is transported throughout the body by the blood.

Air entering the body is—

   21   percent oxygen
   0.04 percent carbon dioxide

The remainder of the air is largely nitrogen.

Air leaving the body is—

   16 percent oxygen
   4 percent carbon dioxide

E. Artificial respiration

Even though there may be doubt as to whether the heart is beating, artificial respiration should be attempted. Artificial respiration does not help if heart action has stopped completely, because then the blood no longer carries oxygen from the lungs to the body cells. Of all the body tissues, cells of the brain are the most sensitive to lack of oxygen. If breathing has stopped and the heart has not been beating for more than from 4 to 6 minutes, the brain is probably permanently damaged to the extent that, even if breathing resumes after this period, the victim might never recover consciousness.

The mouth-to-mouth or mouth-to-nose technique of artificial

respiration, in the absence of equipment, is the most practical method for emergency ventilation of a person of any age who has stopped breathing, regardless of why breathing has stopped. Extensive studies have indicated that mouth-to-mouth and mouth-to-nose resuscitation are unequivocally superior to any of the manual techniques. The mouth-to-mouth or mouth-to-nose technique provides more ventilation than other methods by using direct air pressure exerted by the rescuer to inflate the victim's lungs immediately. It also enables the rescuer to obtain more accurate information on the volume, pressure, and timing of efforts needed to inflate the victim's lungs than is afforded by other methods. Another advantage of this method of artificial respiration, aside from its effectiveness in ventilating the lungs, is that it may be given in the water, in a boat, underneath wreckage, and in other places where immediate resuscitation might be necessary.

The manual methods of artificial respiration are chiefly of historical interest because they are not as effective as the mouth-to-mouth or mouth-to-nose method. The manual methods do not provide as much ventilation as the mouth-to-mouth or mouth-to-nose method, and it is not possible to maintain an open airway at all times when the manual methods are used.

A manual method is not recommended except when the rescuer is unable to perform mouth-to-mouth or mouth-to-nose resuscitation for some reason, such as when massive facial injuries absolutely prevent the use of the mouth-to-mouth or mouth-to-nose method. If a manual method is justified, the preferred method would be the modified Silvester chest pressure-arm lift technique with a support beneath the shoulders to maintain backward tilt of the head. If a second rescuer is present, he should lift the lower jaw or maintain the head in the backward tilt position.

F. Signs and symptoms of respiratory emergencies

Symptoms of respiratory emergencies are characteristic of conditions normally seen in which breathing movements have stopped and there is a lack of oxygen.

1. The victim's tongue, lips, and fingernail beds become blue.

2. There is a loss of consciousness.

3. The pupils become dilated (enlarged).

IV. ARTIFICIAL RESPIRATION

A. Objectives

1. To maintain an open airway through the mouth and nose (or through the stoma)

2. To restore breathing by maintaining an alternating increase and decrease in the expansion of the chest

B. General information

1. The average person may die in 6 minutes or less if his oxygen supply is cut off. It is often impossible to tell *exactly* when a person has stopped breathing; he may be very near death when you first discover him. Therefore, artificial respiration always should be started as rapidly as possible.

2. Recovery is usually rapid except in cases of carbon monoxide poisoning, overdosage of drugs, or electrical shock. In these cases it is often necessary to continue artificial respiration for a long time.

3. When a victim revives, he should be treated for shock. A physician's care is necessary during the recovery period.

4. Artificial respiration should always be continued until—

   a. The victim begins to breathe for himself

   b. He is pronounced dead by a doctor

   c. He is dead beyond any doubt

C. Mouth-to-mouth (mouth-to-nose) method

1. Wipe any obvious foreign matter from the mouth quickly (Fig. 28). Use your fingers, wrapped in a cloth if possible.

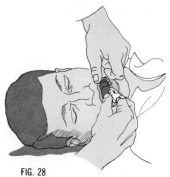

FIG. 28

2. Tilt the victim's head backward so that his chin is pointing upward.

   a. In the unconscious patient in the supine position, the tongue may drop back and block the throat (Fig. 29A). To open the air passage, place one hand beneath the victim's neck and lift. Place the heel of the other hand on the victim's forehead and rotate or tilt his head backward into maximum extension—head-tilt method (Fig. 29B).

   b. For mouth-to-mouth ventilation, maintain the head in this position, since it clears the airway by moving the tongue away from the back of the victim's throat. If additional airway opening is required, it can be achieved by thrusting the lower jaw forward into a jutting-out position—the jaw-thrust method (Fig. 29C).

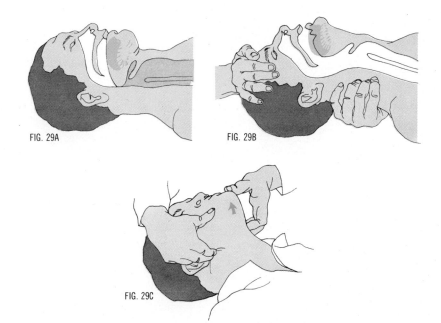

FIG. 29A

FIG. 29B

FIG. 29C

3. Pinch the victim's nostrils shut with the thumb and index finger of your hand that is pressing on the victim's forehead (Fig. 30A). This action prevents leakage of air when the lungs are inflated through the mouth. (Another way is to press your cheek against the victim's nose.)

4. Blow air into the victim's mouth.

    a. Open your mouth widely.

    b. Take a deep breath.

    c. Seal your mouth tightly around the victim's mouth and, with your mouth forming a wide-open circle, blow into his mouth (Fig. 30B).

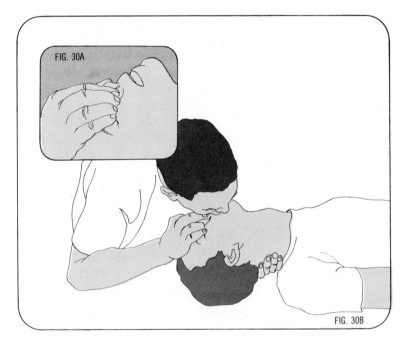

FIG. 30A

FIG. 30B

    d. Provide sufficient air. Volume is important. Start at a high rate and then provide at least one breath every 5 seconds for adults (or 12 per minute).

    e. If the airway is clear, only moderate resistance to blowing will be felt.

5. Watch the victim's chest to see when it rises.

6. Stop blowing when the victim's chest is expanded; raise your mouth; turn your head to the side and listen for exhalation (Fig. 31).

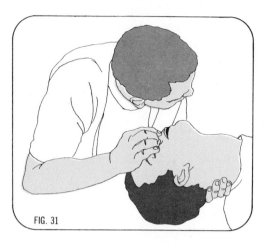

FIG. 31

7. Watch the chest to see that it falls.

8. Repeat the blowing cycle.

9. For the mouth-to-nose method, maintain the backward head tilt position with the hand on the victim's forehead. Use your other hand to close the victim's mouth (Fig. 32A). Open your mouth widely, take a deep breath, seal your mouth tightly around the victim's nose, and blow into the victim's nose (Fig. 32B). On the exhalation phase,

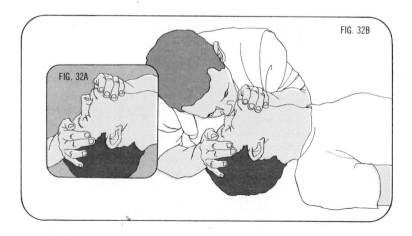

FIG. 32B

FIG. 32A

open the victim's mouth to allow air to escape (Fig. 33).
NOTE. Small children and infants are administered mouth-to-mouth or mouth-to-nose resuscitation as described above, except that the backward head tilt should not be as extensive as that for adults or large children.

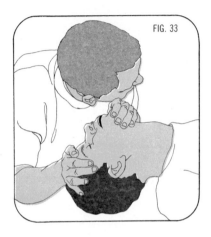

FIG. 33

Both mouth and nose of the infant or small child should be sealed off by your mouth (Fig. 34). Blow into the child's mouth and nose every 3 seconds (about 20 breaths per minute) with less pressure and volume than used for an

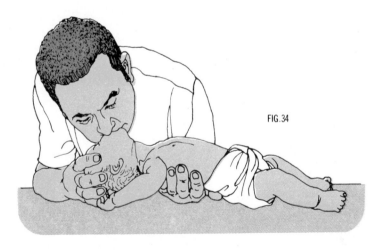

FIG. 34

adult, the amount determined by the size of the child. Only small puffs of air will suffice for infants.

10. If you are not getting air exchange, recheck the position of the head and jaw and check to see if there is foreign matter in the back of the mouth that may be obstructing the air passage.

    If still unable to ventilate, seek a foreign body that may be deep in the airway, causing obstruction. Insert the index and middle fingers of one hand inside the victim's cheek and slide them deeply into the throat to the base of the tongue. Use a sweeping motion to carry them through the back of the throat and out along the inside of the other cheek to try to remove the foreign body.

11. If foreign matter is preventing ventilation, as a last resort, turn the victim on his side and administer sharp blows between the shoulder blades to jar the material free (Fig. 35).

    A child may be suspended momentarily by the ankles or turned upside down over one arm and given two or three sharp blows between the shoulder blades (Fig. 36).

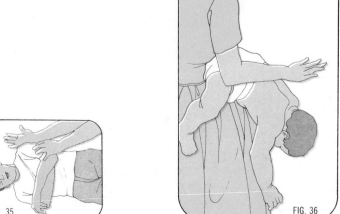

FIG. 36

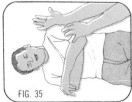

FIG. 35

12. Clear the mouth again, reposition, and repeat mouth-to-mouth or mouth-to-nose respiration.

If the victim's stomach is bulging, air may have been blown into the stomach, particularly when the air passage is obstructed or the inflation pressure is excessive. Although inflation of the stomach is not dangerous, it may make lung ventilation more difficult and increase the likelihood of vomiting.

If the stomach is bulging, always turn the victim's head to one side and be prepared to clear the mouth before pressing your hand briefly and firmly over the upper abdomen, between the rib margin and the navel (Fig. 37). This

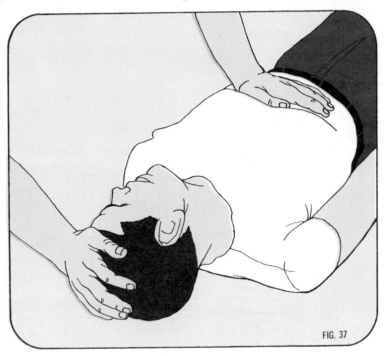

FIG. 37

procedure will force air out of the stomach but it may also cause regurgitation.

Some persons who require artificial respiration never stop breathing completely but gasp irregularly. Efforts toward breathing assist in recovery but they should not encourage you to abandon mouth-to-mouth resuscitation until a normal pattern of respiration has been restored. Coordinate your blowing with the victim's inhalation.

D. Mouth-to-stoma method

1. The laryngectomee

   In the United States there are about 25,000 persons whose larynxes have been completely or partially removed by surgery. The operation is called a *laryngectomy*. Those who have had the operation are called *laryngectomees* (Fig. 38).

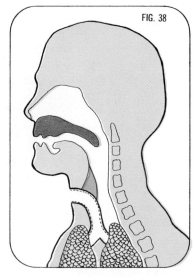

FIG. 38

A laryngectomee breathes through an opening called a *stoma* in the windpipe (trachea) in front of the neck; he cannot use his nose or mouth for breathing.

2. First aid for laryngectomees

   a. When examining a victim of an accident or sudden illness, check the front of the neck to determine if the victim is a laryngectomee. (Most laryngectomees carry a card or other identification stating that they cannot breathe through the nose or mouth.)

   b. Do not inadvertently block the stoma when carrying out other first aid.

   The sound of escaping air, especially in combination

with secretions or blood flow after injury in the neck area, may mislead the first-aider to conclude that the injury constitutes a sucking wound of the chest (see page 81) and he may thus attempt to block the stoma with a pressure dressing. Blockage must be avoided, since it could cause death from asphyxiation.

c. If a person is wearing a breathing tube in the stoma, leave it in place unless it becomes clogged by foreign material, causing breathing difficulties.

If the laryngectomee is conscious, he may want to clean the tube and replace it himself, and he should be permitted to do so. Otherwise, the first-aider should send the tube with the victim to the hospital for replacement in the stoma.

d. Give artificial respiration using the same general procedure as for mouth-to-mouth resuscitation, but place your mouth firmly over the victim's stoma. Blow at the same rate as for a person who breathes normally, watching the victim's chest for inflow of air (Fig. 39).

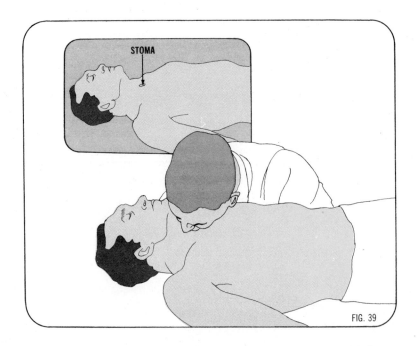

FIG. 39

    (1) Keep the victim's head straight. It is not necessary to tilt the head backward and to close off the victim's nose and mouth.

    (2) Avoid twisting the victim's head. Twisting might change the shape of, or close, the stoma.

    (3) Do not be concerned with the victim's tongue or dentures blocking his airway.

    (4) It is possible that the laryngectomy may be partial instead of complete, in which case the person breathes both through the stoma and the mouth and nose. If the stoma is clear and the victim's chest does not rise when the first-aider blows through the stoma, tilt the victim's head back, close off the mouth and nose, and continue the blowing efforts through the stoma.

  3. Advantages of the mouth-to-stoma method

    a. The mouth-to-stoma method is more sanitary than mouth-to-mouth resuscitation because air coming from the stoma is cleaner than air coming from the mouth. Also, the contents of the laryngectomee's stomach cannot be vomited into the first-aider's mouth, because there is no connection between the stomach and the stoma.

    b. The mouth-to-stoma method is preferred over a manual method since it is much more effective. The use of the Silvester method is justified only when the only first-aider available is also a laryngectomee. If the manual method is used, make sure to keep the victim's head straight.

E. Chest pressure-arm lift method (Silvester method)

  1. If foreign matter is visible in the victim's mouth, wipe it out quickly with your fingers, preferably with a cloth wrapped around them.

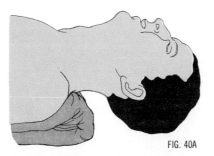

FIG. 40A

  2. Place the victim in a face-up position. Maintain an open airway. An open airway can be maintained by placing something under the victim's shoulders to raise them several inches and allowing his head to drop backward (Fig. 40A). Turn his head to the side.

3. Kneel at the top of the victim's head, grasp his wrists, and cross them over his lower chest (Fig. 40B).

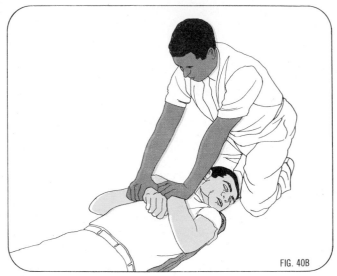

FIG. 40B

4. Rock forward until your arms are approximately vertical and allow the weight of the upper part of your body to exert steady, even pressure downward (Fig. 41). This action will cause air to flow out of the victim's chest.

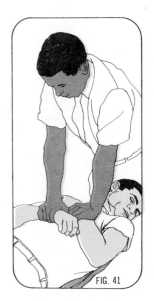

FIG. 41

5. Immediately release the pressure by rocking back, pulling the victim's arms outward and upward over his head and backward as far as possible (Fig. 42A). This procedure should cause air to flow in.

6. Repeat this cycle about 12 times per minute, checking the victim's mouth often for obstruction.

7. There is always danger of aspirating vomitus, blood, or blood clots. This hazard can be reduced by keeping the victim's head a little lower than his trunk. A helper should pull the victim's jaw forward and up and be alert to detect the presence of any stomach contents in the victim's mouth (Fig. 42B). The victim's mouth should be kept as clean as possible at all times. Remove any airway obstruction, as described in the technique for mouth-to-mouth breathing.

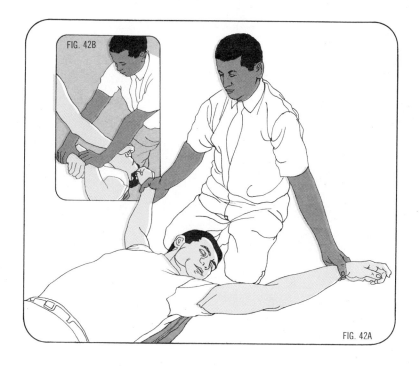

FIG. 42B

FIG. 42A

V. CARDIOPULMONARY RESUSCITATION

Cardiopulmonary resuscitation (CPR) is the combination of artificial respiration and manual artificial circulation that is recommended for use in cases of cardiac arrest. It requires special supplemental training in the recognition of cardiac arrest and in the performance of CPR. Instruction includes manikin practice in performing both individually and as part of a team. Periodic retraining is required unless rescuers have repeated experiences in the application of CPR.

Cardiopulmonary resuscitation should be carried out only by qualified persons.

A. General Procedure

Cardiopulmonary resuscitation involves the following steps:
A—Airway opening
B—Breathing restored
C—Circulation restored
D—Definitive therapy

External cardiac compression consists of the application of rhythmic pressure over the lower half of the sternum. This pressure compresses the heart and produces a pulsatile artificial circulation. External cardiac compression must always be accompanied by artificial ventilation.

B. Definitive therapy

Definitive therapy involves diagnosis, drugs, defibrillation (when indicated), and disposition. Definitive procedures are restricted to physicians or to members of allied health professions and authorized paramedical personnel under medical direction. The recommended basic techniques for performing the A and B steps are clearly defined in this text. The C and D steps are procedures requiring special supplemental training.

VI. PREVENTION OF RESPIRATORY ACCIDENTS

A large number of accidental deaths occur each year because of blockage and stoppage of natural breathing. The material that follows will consider only the most common conditions and activities that produce respiratory emergencies. A better under-

1. Supervision

   Swimming, wading, or playing about in unguarded water is a major causative factor in drownings. A drowning accident often occurs quickly and quietly. Self-protection and the protection of others require both competent and constant supervision. Never swim alone, and stay away from or out of the water unless proper supervision is provided.

2. Protection

   Residential pools, particularly at homes, pose an accident problem of growing concern to neighbors, communities, and public safety officials. Aside from the common-sense protective measures of constant and competent supervision when such pools are in use, protection against trespassers or unsuspecting toddlers also deserves concerted attention.

   Around residential pools, install an enclosure designed to prevent or discourage trespassers and small children from unauthorized entry. The fact that such enclosures may not be required by law in some communities should not keep residential pool owners from meeting this protective necessity.

   Another protective consideration involves the availability and use of simple rescue devices around residential-type pools and swimming ponds. A reaching pole is an example of such an item and is one of the basic rescue devices that anyone can learn to use.

   Open wells, cisterns, and water-filled excavations also present a water accident hazard. Wells and cisterns can often be capped to prevent accidental entry. Fencing is sometimes a more practical solution, particularly in the case of water-filled excavations that cannot be pumped and kept dry.

3. Training

   Water safety training should begin at a very young age. The danger of prolonged submersion can be learned by many children at the age of 3 or 4. The ages of 5 through 8 offer an opportune time for most youngsters to begin

standing of how such respiratory accidents can be pr(
develop when all possible circumstances surrounding \
accident types are considered and discussed.

A. Drowning accidents

Drowning accidents are the fourth leading cause of .
tal death. In the active age groups, drowning ranks se
fatalities only to motor vehicle accidents. The majo
fatal water accidents occur in the pursuit of recreation;
or leisure-time activities.

More than half of all drownings happen to people who u
pectedly find themselves in the water. Boating accidents
a prime example. Careless operation, overpowering of mot
boats, overloading, bad weather, dangerous water conditioi
and irresponsible behavior of a craft's occupants are commo
causes of such accidents. Other nonswimming fatalities in
volve persons falling into the water while fishing, working, or
merely playing on docks, bridges, and shorelines, and cases of
children tumbling into open wells, cisterns, water-filled excavations, and unprotected swimming pools.

Wading or swimming in unguarded water also results in a
great many drownings. A cry for help may well prove futile
to the wading victim of a river-bottom hole, open water drop-
off, or strong current that sweeps him off his feet, or to an
exhausted swimmer who overestimated his swimming ability
in unguarded water.

A knowledge of hazardous conditions and practices, and good
skill ability are basic to an individual's safety while in, on, or
about the water.

Inability to swim is a contributing cause in most accidental
drownings. Regardless of the water sport or activity, training
in swimming skills and knowledge is essential to safe enjoyment.

Prevention of accidental drownings, therefore, involves supervision, protection, and training. Other factors may enter
into a water accident prevention program, but these are the
main components.

receiving formal swimming instruction. Training in the operation of small craft and other water recreational activities likewise can begin at an early age.

Basic water safety education should begin in the home environment. While parents can help a young child develop a sensible regard for the hazards of water, the parents must be careful that such efforts do not destroy the child's desire to enjoy the water. Water safety education may best be accomplished when formal instruction for swimming or any special water sport activity is placed with agencies properly designated and equipped to meet such educational responsibility—such as the Coast Guard, the Red Cross, schools, and community groups.

Take advantage of swimming, lifesaving, small craft, and other formal aquatic training programs in your community. If none exist, find out what it takes to get them going and then support efforts to do so.

B. Ingested and inhaled objects

A frequent cause of respiratory blockage, especially with very young children, is swallowed or inhaled food and physical objects that can lodge in the throat.

Protect infants and teething toddlers from swallowing small objects and food particles large enough to require chewing. (For specific accident prevention information, see chapter 6.)

C. Mechanical suffocation

Respiratory emergencies in the home are mainly the result of mechanical suffocation from smothering, strangulation, and closed-space confinement. Mechanical suffocation is the leading cause of accidental death to infants under 1 year of age. Suffocation can occur when the child is smothered by bedclothing, thin plastic wrapping materials, or plastic mattress covers—or even the body of a sleeping parent or older child. It can also result from strangulation by an item such as a venetian blind cord.

Control shifting and bunching of bedclothing. Never give an infant thin plastic material to play with, and be certain that plastic mattress covers are securely anchored to the mattress. Recognize the danger of allowing an infant to sleep in a bed alongside a larger person. Place an infant's crib away from windows where venetian blind cords may come in contact with the child.

D. Gas inhalation and electric current

Carbon monoxide gas is a natural by-product of the incomplete combustion of many fuels and most open fires. As this gas is breathed, it replaces oxygen in the blood. When oxygen in the blood reaches a critically low level, the breathing mechanism in the brain fails, and breathing stops.

Conditions that allow carbon monoxide to accumulate in closed spaces should be eliminated. Do not, for example, run a motor vehicle in a closed garage. Vent all heating equipment to the outside, and be certain the venting pipe is always free of soot and other obstructions. Avoid entering enclosed areas where carbon monoxide gas is suspected or known to exist, such as a smoke-filled room. If you must enter a room where carbon monoxide gas is present, remember that the only uncontaminated air that will be available until your exit is the air inhaled outside the room; the breath must be held until you exit from the contaminated room. Nothing but a proper gas mask will afford protection if inhalation must occur within a gas-filled room.

Workers employed in occupations where poisonous gas, vapors, or smoke can be encountered, or in environments underground, underwater, or at altitudes where oxygen can be limited or absent, must take special precautions against potential respiratory failure. Protective masks and an auxiliary supply of contained oxygen are necessary protective devices in such hazardous working conditions.

Electric current that reaches or passes through the body also creates a danger of respiratory failure. This hazard is discussed under "Fires of Electrical Origin," page 155.

VII. SWIMMING SAFETY TIPS

A. Prevention and precautions

Everyone should learn how to swim at an early age. Red Cross chapters and other groups offer swimming instructions in communities throughout the nation. In addition, everyone should know and observe these basic rules.

1. Never swim alone; make sure there is someone nearby who can help in an emergency.

2. Adjust slowly to cool or cold water; do not plunge in.

3. Swim at a safe swimming place, preferably one supervised by lifeguards.

4. Beware of unfamiliar swimming areas, since they may have treacherous currents, deep holes, debris, and other hazards.

5. Do not swim when overheated or overtired, or immediately after eating a heavy meal or even a meal of normal size.

6. Before diving, make sure that the water is deep enough and has no hidden objects beneath the surface. Do not dive into a swimming pool without checking first to make sure that the water is deep enough for diving and that there are no swimmers beneath you.

7. Know your own ability and do not overestimate it; judging distance accurately over water is difficult.

8. When swimming underwater, come up to the surface as soon as your chest is tight and you feel that you need air.

9. If you are planning on a distance swim in open water, have someone accompany you in a boat.

10. Be courteous; consider the safety of others.

11. Do not duck anyone or hold his head underwater.

12. Do not push anyone into the water.

B. Water safety for small children

1. Never leave a baby or small child alone in the bathtub or in a wading pool, even for a few seconds.

2. If you have a fishpond or swimming pool, to protect small children, put a fence around it that cannot be climbed easily and equip the gate with a safety lock.

3. Warn children about playing near canals, ponds, quarries, irrigation ditches, and the like.

4. Teach children how to swim at an early age.

5. Make sure that young children wear life jackets when they are playing around pools or other water.

6. Do not allow children to use water wings, tires, or other inflated objects to float in deep water or alone in the surf.

VIII. BOATING SAFETY TIPS

A. Learn to swim and to handle your craft properly and safely. Carry emergency equipment. Many Red Cross chapters and other groups offer courses in canoeing, sailing, outboard motorboating, and rowing.

B. Learn the nautical rules of the road.

C. Have a Coast Guard approved personal flotation device for each person on board your boat.

D. In small watercraft, children and weak swimmers should wear a flotation device at all times.

E. If you are using an outboard motor, match the motor to the boat. Do not overload your boat. Overloading is dangerous. Follow the capacity rating for your boat.

F. Keep your weight low in the craft at all times. Do not stand up in small boats.

G. If bad weather is threatening, do not go out. If the weather gets rough, return to shore, or seek shelter away from wind and waves.

H. If your canoe or small boat upsets or fills with water, it will usually float. Hold onto it for support or enter it and sit in the bottom. Even with the motor attached, the boat will probably support the normal number of occupants.

I. Whenever you go out in a boat, in case of an emergency, leave word with family members or marina personnel on where you plan to go and when you expect to return.

6

SWALLOWED OBJECTS AND CHOKING

Each year nearly 2,000 deaths occur in the United States due to asphyxia caused by obstruction of breathing. Two-thirds of the deaths reported apply to children under the age of 4.

I. CAUSES

    A. A small child investigates an object by placing it into his mouth.

    B. A child cannot chew well until dentition is sufficient.

    C. An inedible substance can become caught in the throat.

    D. Objects can be aspirated into lower air passages.

    E. Obstruction may occur in adults when swallowing unchewed meat or food containing splinters of bone or shell.

    F. Persons with dentures are prone to choke on food, since normal chewing sensation is diminished.

    G. Eating without dentures is hazardous.

    H. Alcoholic beverages before a meal decrease sensation in the mouth and normal vigilance and caution in eating, thus increasing the danger of choking.

II. SIGNS AND SYMPTOMS

    A. Violent choking

    B. Alarming attempts at inhalation (stridor or crowing sounds)

    C. Discoloration (cyanosis) of the face, neck, and hands

D. Cessation of breathing

E. Unconsciousness

III. FIRST AID

The objective of first aid for a person who is choking is to allow the victim to assume a comfortable position and encourage him to cough. If breathing fails, administer artificial respiration and, if necessary, attempt to expel the object. Obtain immediate medical attention.

A. Swallowed objects in food passages

1. Give nothing by mouth until advised by a physician.

2. Do not give any cathartic or laxative drug to a person who has swallowed a foreign object.

3. If the object is small and not sharp, observe the victim's feces to determine whether the object has passed safely through the digestive tract.

4. Remove a foreign object that is accessible to your fingers but take great care in removing it. A foreign object lodged in the back of the victim's throat should not be removed with your fingers, because either the pressure on the object or the swallowing efforts may force the object more deeply into the victim's throat.

B. Aspiration of fluids and objects in the larynx or lower air passages

A foreign body aspirated into the air passages creates an immediate crisis. Foreign bodies are usually trapped by a spasm of the muscles at the level of the larynx. The victim is unable to breathe for a few seconds. The spasm then relaxes, and the object often will be coughed out. Coughing is a protective mechanism by which a foreign body is sometimes expelled from the larynx.

1. If the object cannot be expelled by the victim within a moment or so, seek medical help at once.

2. Allow the victim to assume a position most comfortable for him.

3. Do not attempt to remove the object with your fingers.

4. Encourage the victim to cough as soon as the spasm of the larynx subsides.

5. Remain calm and reassure the victim.

6. Do not give cough syrup, medicines, crackers, or bread.

C. Foreign body prohibiting ventilation

Artificial respiration should be administered only if the victim ceases to breathe or if breathing is ineffectual and death appears imminent. If unable to ventilate, seek a foreign body that may be deep in the airway, causing obstruction. Insert the index and middle fingers of one hand inside the victim's cheek and slide them deeply into the throat to the base of the tongue. Use a sweeping motion to carry them through the back of the throat and out along the inside of the other cheek to try to remove the foreign body.

As a last resort, the first-aider should attempt to move the object blocking the air passages by turning the adult victim onto his side and using the heel of the hand to administer sharp blows between the shoulder blades over the spine. A child may be turned upside down over one arm and given two or three sharp blows between the shoulder blades. Even though relief is obtained, the victim should receive medical attention after an episode of choking.

IV. PREVENTION

A. For small children

1. Keep articles that may be accidentally swallowed or aspirated out of the reach of infants and small children.

2. Caution older children not to put small objects in a baby's mouth or within his reach.

3. Do not hold open safety pins in the mouth when changing a baby's diaper. A pin may slip out of the mother's mouth into the mouth of the infant. Take care not to leave safety pins within reach of the child.

4. Provide sturdy, safe toys without small parts that might become detached.

5. Do not give small children nuts or candy containing nuts,

raw carrots or other uncooked vegetables, fruits that require chewing, unchopped meat, or any foods containing seeds or pits until the age of 4.

6. Do not allow a child to play with beans, peas, hard kernels of corn, or large seeds.

7. Do not stimulate a child to laugh or cry when he has food in his mouth.

8. Do not permit a child to run about while eating.

9. Remove bones and shells from all foods given to a child.

10. As soon as he is old enough to learn, teach a child not to put foreign objects in his mouth.

B. For older children and adults

1. Eat slowly; chew food thoroughly; watch for small particles of bone, seed, or shell. Cut meat into small pieces.

2. Prepare food carefully; watch for foreign objects in the kitchen that may become mixed with food.

3. If you are choking, remain calm. Wait until the spasm passes and then cough hard. Do not try to talk.

4. If you wear dentures, take special precautions in eating. Keep them in good repair. Do not wear defective dentures at night.

5. Do not go to sleep with chewing gum in your mouth.

6. Do not chew on objects that may be swallowed or aspirated. Aside from the danger, the practice sets a bad example for small children, who learn by imitation.

7. Do not assume that all is well if symptoms disappear. Consult a physician after an episode of choking unless the object has been definitely expelled. Make a note in a diary. Infection may develop later in the lung.

8. Do not allow anyone to slap you on your back if you choke and do not try to dislodge an object from another person's throat by this means, except as a last, desperate effort to save his life.

7

POISONING

I. DEFINITION

A poison is any substance, solid, liquid, or gas, that tends to impair health, or cause death, when introduced into the body or onto the skin surface.

II. CAUSES

Small children are especially likely to become poisoning victims since they tend to put into their mouths nearly everything that they pick up. However, adults are subject to poisoning also.

A. Frequent causes of poisoning

1. Overdoses of aspirin, especially in children

2. Medicines left within reach of children

3. Poisons transferred from the original containers to jars or soft drink bottles

4. Carelessness on the part of parents in leaving dangerous substances around, particularly when children cannot yet read

5. Lack of supervision

6. Improper storage and disposal of poisonous substances

7. Improper handling of spray equipment, including the mixing of pesticides, insecticides, and weed killers

8. Inhalation or swallowing of poisonous substances

9. Carelessness in taking a poison from the medicine cabinet

10. Overdoses of drugs, done either accidentally or with suicidal intent

11. Combining drugs and alcohol

B. Examples of poisons around the home

Poisonous substances within the home environment are extremely prevalent, and it would be difficult to name all of them. A few typical household poisons are listed below:

1. Cosmetics, hair preparations

2. Gasoline, kerosene, and other petroleum products

3. Paint and turpentine

4. Strong detergents

5. Bleaches

6. Cleaning solutions

7. Lye

8. Glue

9. Ammonia

10. Acids

11. Poisonous plants, such as mountain laurel, rhododendron, oleander, a variety of wild cherries, nightshade, and fox glove

12. Nonedible mushrooms

C. Ways in which poisoning may occur

1. By mouth

2. By absorption

3. By inhalation

4. By injection

III. SIGNS AND SYMPTOMS

Symptoms of poisoning vary greatly. Aids in determining whether or not a victim has swallowed poison include—

A. Information from the victim or from an observer

B. Presence of a container known to contain poison

C. Condition of the victim (sudden onset of pain or illness)

D. Burns around the lips or mouth

E. Breath odor

F. Pupils of the eyes contracted to pinpoint size from an over-dose of morphine or similar drugs

IV. OBJECTIVES IN TREATMENT OF POISONING BY MOUTH

The objectives in treatment of poisoning by mouth are to dilute or neutralize the poison as quickly as possible, to induce vomiting (except when corrosive poisons are swallowed or if victim is unconscious or having convulsions), to maintain respiration, to preserve vital functions, and to seek medical assistance without delay.

V. FIRST AID

Begin immediately to carry out the above objectives as quickly as possible.

WHAT TO DO WHEN—

You do know that the victim has not swallowed a strong acid, strong alkali, or petroleum product, but do not have the original container.	You do not know what poison the victim swallowed.
1. Dilute the poison with water or milk.	1. Dilute the poison with water or milk.
2. Induce vomiting (except for strong acids, strong alkalis, and petroleum products).	2. Try to find out what poison has been swallowed. (Look for the original container.)
3. Get medical help immediately.	3. Get medical help immediately.

A. If the victim is unconscious, keep his airway open; give him artificial respiration if indicated; transport him as quickly as possible to receive medical help. Take along the poison container or a sample of vomitus if available. Do not give fluids to an unconscious victim.

B. Whenever possible, have someone else get advice by telephoning a doctor, a hospital emergency room, or a poison control information center, while you are giving first aid to the victim. The caller should telephone for an ambulance and the police if there is an indication of suicide or homicide. If assistance is not available, give vital first aid immediately, and, as quickly as possible, obtain medical advice. Give the following information:

   1. Age of the victim

   2. Name of the poison and amount taken, if known; otherwise, the general nature of the drug or chemical

   3. First aid being given

   4. Whether or not the victim has vomited

   5. Your location and the time it will take to get to the physician or the hospital, and whether police escort will be necessary

C. If a specific antidote is described on the label of a commercial product, administer it according to directions if the victim is conscious.

D. Give, if available a commercial preparation called the universal antidote, which contains medicinal charcoal as its most important ingredient.

E. Save the label or container for identification of the poison, also a sample of the vomited material if available.

F. Estimate the amount taken from the amount remaining in the container (if any).

G. If a person has taken tranquilizers, barbiturates, paregoric, opium-containing drugs, or alcohol, give him coffee or strong tea as a stimulant if he is conscious. (Also see chapter 8.)

H. If the victim is having convulsions, *do not* give any medications and do not induce vomiting. Arrange transportation as quickly as possible.

1. Do not attempt to restrain the victim, but position him in such a manner that he will not injure himself by knocking against furniture or other objects.

2. Loosen tight clothing at the victim's neck and waist.

3. Do not force a hard object or your finger between the victim's teeth.

4. Watch for an obstruction of the victim's airway. Give artificial respiration if indicated.

5. Do not give anything to drink.

I. After the convulsions, turn the victim on his side, or face down with his head turned to one side, so that mucus will drain from his mouth.

J. In most cases of oral poisoning, induce vomiting as soon as you have given the victim water or milk. Vomiting can be induced by tickling the back of the victim's throat with your finger or by giving him a nauseating fluid, such as syrup of ipecac or mustard and water.

K. Whenever a poisoning victim vomits, whether you caused it or not, position the victim on his side or stomach (hold a small child on your lap) with his head lower than his hips so that the vomited poison will not reenter the food and breathing passages.

L. In some poisoning cases, vomiting should not be induced. Vomiting a strong acid, such as toilet bowl cleaner, or a strong alkali, such as drain cleaner, can cause further burns in air and food passages that have already been burned. Vomiting a petroleum product, such as gasoline, kerosene, or furniture polish, can cause pneumonia.

M. The signs that tell you *not* to induce vomiting are—

1. Burns around the lips and mouth

2. Breath odor (kerosene or gasoline, for example)

3. Information on the container

4. Unconsciousness

5. Convulsions

6. Exhaustion

N. *Do not* dilute fluid or induce vomiting when the victim is unconscious, having convulsions, or suffering from exhaustion. In these three cases, keep the victim quiet and warm, and get medical help immediately.

O. Except as noted above, immediately give a poisoning victim water or milk to dilute the poison. In addition to diluting the poison, you may find it necessary to administer a neutralizer and a demulcent (soothing substance with coating action). A demulcent tends to coat the lining of the stomach and intestines, and helps to slow down the absorption of a poison. Milk, olive oil, and egg whites are demulcents.

P. After diluting the poison and giving a neutralizer and a demulcent, you should call a doctor or take the victim immediately to the nearest hospital.

Q. A neutralizer, which may be thought of as the chemical opposite the nature of the poison, tends to reduce the poison's harmful effects. For example, a weak acid, such as lemon juice or vinegar, tends to neutralize a strong alkali, such as drain cleaner. A weak alkali, such as milk of magnesia, tends to neutralize a strong acid, such as toilet bowl cleaner.

R. The following table illustrates the order and the type of fluids to be administered to a poisoning victim when vomiting should *not* be induced.

S. <u>First aid</u> for inhaled poison gases

Carbon monoxide, the most common poisonous gas, formed from incomplete burning of fuel, is particularly treacherous since it is completely odorless. The victim may lose consciousness and be asphyxiated with no warning symptoms other than slight dizziness, weakness, and headache. Death may occur in a few minutes, thus necessitating quick action. The victim's lips and skin are characteristically a cherry red.

1. If the victim is in a closed room, garage, or other small space, take a deep breath and hold it before entering. Remove the victim to a source of fresh air, if possible; otherwise, call the fire department or a rescue squad.

2. Maintain an open airway.

3. Give artificial respiration, if indicated.

4. Loosen tight clothing.

5. Seek medical assistance as quickly as possible. Indicate the nature of the problem and that oxygen should be brought to the scene.

TYPES OF POISONS FOR WHICH VOMITING
SHOULD NOT BE INDUCED

Type of Poison	Diluting Fluids (One glass)	Neutralizing Fluid (Adult: 3-4 glasses) (Child: 1-2 glasses)	Demulcent (Several glasses but do not cause vomiting)
Strong acid (for example, toilet bowl cleaner)	Water or milk	Milk of magnesia or other weak alkali, mixed with water	Milk, olive oil, or egg white
Strong alkali (for example, drain cleaner)	Water or milk	Vinegar or lemon juice, mixed with water	Milk, olive oil, or egg white
Petroleum product (for example, kerosene, gasoline, furniture polish)	Water or milk	None	None

VI. CONTACT POISONS

A. Chemical burns

Harsh chemicals and corrosive poisons, if spilled on the skin, produce chemical burns, which require immediate first aid (see chapter 9).

B. Contact with poisonous plants

1. Characteristic reactions

   The majority of skin reactions following contact with offending plants are allergic in nature and are characterized by—

   a. General symptoms of headache and fever

   b. Itching

   c. Redness

   d. A rash

   Some of the most common and most severe allergic reactions result from contact with plants of the poison ivy group (Fig. 43), including poison oak and poison sumac. Such plants produce severe rash characterized by redness, blisters, swelling, and intense burning and itching. The victim also may develop a high fever and may be very ill. Ordinarily, the rash begins within a few hours after exposure, but it may be delayed for from 24 to 48 hours.

2. Distinguishing features of poison ivy group plants
   The most distinctive features of poison ivy and poison oak are their leaves, which are composed of three leaflets each. Both plants also have greenish-white flowers and berries that grow in clusters.

3. First aid

   a. Remove contaminated clothing; wash all exposed areas thoroughly with soap and water, followed by rubbing alcohol.

   b. Apply calamine or other soothing skin lotion if the rash is mild.

   c. Seek medical advice if a severe reaction occurs, or if there is a known history of previous sensitivity.

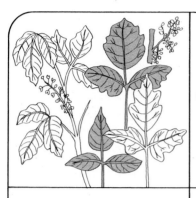

COMMON POISON IVY
(RHUS RADICANS)

• Grows as a small plant, a vine, and a shrub.

• Grows everywhere in the United States except California and parts of adjacent states. Eastern oak leaf poison ivy is one of its varieties.

• Leaves always consist of three glossy leaflets.

• Also known as three-leaf ivy, poison creeper, climbing sumac, poison oak, markweed, picry, and mercury.

WESTERN POISON OAK
(RHUS DIVERSILOBA)

• Grows in shrub and sometimes vine form.

• Grows in California and parts of adjacent states.

• Sometimes called poison ivy, or yeara.

• Leaves always consist of three leaflets.

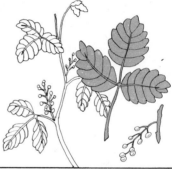

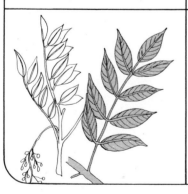

POISON SUMAC
(RHUS VERNIX)

• Grows as a woody shrub or small tree from 5 to 25 feet tall.

• Grows in most of eastern third of United States.

• Also known as swamp sumac, poison elder, poison ash, poison dogwood, and thunderwood.

FIG. 43

C. <u>First aid</u> for contact poisons

    1. Remove the contaminated clothing; immediately drench and flush the affected skin with large quantities of water or other available liquids, as you remove clothing.

    2. If poisoning is from a pesticide or a corrosive substance (strong acid or alkali), send for an ambulance immediately.

    3. Continue washing all contaminated skin with soap and water for at least 5 minutes.

    4. Keep the victim's airway open. Give artificial respiration if indicated. Do not leave the victim alone.

VII. PREVENTION

A. Prevention of poisoning from drugs and chemicals

    1. Storage

Store all household chemical products and medicines out of reach and sight of children, preferably in a locked cabinet or closet. Medicines and chemicals should not be stored on shelves with food. Label them properly.

Keep medicines, chemicals, and cosmetic preparations in their original containers. Do not transfer poisonous products to unlabeled bottles, glasses, or cups. Do not reuse containers that have held potentially harmful substances.

    2. Use

Read labels before taking medicines. Do not take or give medicine at night without turning on the light.

Protect your skin and eyes when using insect poisons, weed killers, solvents, strong detergents, and cleaning agents. Use liquids and sprays only in well-ventilated places. Wear a mask over your mouth and nose when spraying paints, pesticides, and similar preparations. Do not use gasoline or kerosene for starting fires or for cleaning purposes. Wash thoroughly after using strong chemicals and remove contaminated clothing at once. Clean up any spilled liquid.

    3. Precautions to observe around children

Avoid taking medicine in the presence of small children. Safeguard, with special precautions, all drugs that are colored, flavored, or coated with sugar (including aspirin-containing chewing gum). Warn small children not to eat or drink medicines or anything else they may find without your permission. Insist upon this rule as soon as they are old enough to begin exploring the home environment.

Teach children about the danger of drugs and poisonous chemicals. Do not allow them to inhale plastic glues or resins for a prolonged period of time while building plastic models. Provide teenagers with information regarding the dangers of drinking industrial alcohols, overdoses of alcohol, and experimentation with drugs.

4. Disposal

Take an inventory of drugs and chemicals in the home. Discard old drugs periodically, particularly those left over from treatment of special illnesses. Flush the drugs down the drain. Rinse containers and throw them away.

5. Preparation for emergencies

Learn what to do in case of overdose of medication or accidental poisoning. Keep first aid supplies on hand and available at all times. Also keep handy the telephone numbers of your physician, hospital, and poison control information center and the police and fire departments.

B. Prevention of poisoning from plants

1. Ingested poisons

Prevention of poisoning in small children depends upon early training *not* to chew on leaves or plants or to eat berries that they may find, without permission. Adults, particularly those on farms and with gardens, should learn which plants are likely to produce poisoning if swallowed accidentally or included, by chance, with edible vegetables and berries.

2. Contact with poisonous plants

Learn to identify the poisonous plants in locations where you live and visit. Persons with known sensitivity should avoid contact with noxious plants or consult their physicians regarding desensitization injections.

Since poisonous plants often are not recognized as such, or are identified only after contact, all persons who have been handling wild flowers, leaves, and plants should remove contaminated clothing and thoroughly wash exposed surfaces of the skin as soon as possible.

Stay away from irritating plants that are being burned, since the soot may contain active substances that produce a reaction. The toxic extract also may be transmitted by pets and from clothing.

VIII. POISONING BY MARINE LIFE

A. Causes and effects

1. Marine animals can produce puncture wounds.

2. Toxic reactions may result in varying effects due to individual sensitivity or resistance and the virulence and amount of venom inflicted or contacted.

3. A variety of species of fish are equipped with venom apparatus attached to dorsal or other spines. A few examples are—

   a. Catfish

   b. Weever fish

   c. Scorpion fish (including zebrafish)

   d. Toadfish and surgeonfish

   First aid treatment relates to the symptom, since little is known regarding antidotes.

4. Seasnakes, uncommon in water bordering the United States, are of the cobra genus and inject extremely potent venom that affects the nervous system. First aid is the same as for other snakebites.

B. Ingestion of poisonous shellfish and fish

1. Characteristics

   Shellfish poisoning, while unpredictable, is more common from March to November than during the rest of the year. Shellfish poisoning is related to—

a. Bacterial contamination

b. Allergic reactions

c. A paralytic type of poison due to ingestion by clams and mussels of microscopic, poisonous, marine animals called Dinoflagellates

   (1) Symptoms of paralytic-type poisoning

      (a) Numbness of the face and mouth

      (b) Weakness

      (c) Muscular paralysis

      (d) Increased salivation

      (e) Intense thirst

      (f) Difficulty in swallowing

   (2) Location

     The poison is concentrated in the dark meat, gills, digestive organs, and siphon of the shellfish.

2. Precautions

There are numerous varieties of shellfish that should not be eaten. Learn the species of marine life in your area that are known to be safe.

3. First aid

First aid for ingestion of fish and for shellfish poisoning is the same as for noncorrosive poisons:

a. Induce vomiting.

b. Dilute poison.

c. Treat for shock.

d. Give artificial respiration if indicated.

e. Individuals having allergic reactions to scombroid fish (for example, mackerel) or shellfish should seek medical advice regarding the administration of an antihistamine.

C. Stings

1. From jellyfish and the Portuguese man-of-war

a. Characteristics

Jellyfish (Fig. 44A) and the Portuguese man-of-war (Fig. 44B) have stinging cells (Fig. 44C), located on

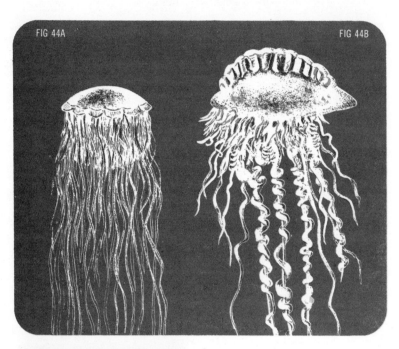

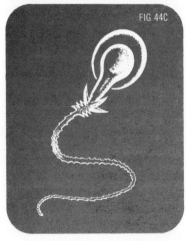

their tentacles, that discharge venom through thread-like tubes upon contact. The venom produces—

(1) Burning pain

(2) A rash with minute hemorrhages in the skin

(3) Shock on occasion

(4) Muscular cramping

(5) Nausea and vomiting

(6) Respiratory difficulty

b. <u>First aid</u>

(1) Wipe off the affected area with a towel, and wash the area thoroughly with diluted ammonia or rubbing alcohol.

(2) Give home medication, such as aspirin, for pain.

(3) Seek medical aid if symptoms are severe.

2. From stinging coral (Fig. 45)

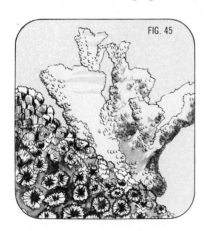

FIG. 45

a. Characteristics and precautions

Stinging coral (fire coral) inject venom through stinging cells, producing multiple sharp cuts, contaminated by particles of broken-off calcareous (calcium-containing) material. All workers around coral should wear gloves, flippers or canvas shoes, and an outergarment for protection.

b. <u>First aid</u>

(1) Clean thoroughly.

(2) Seek prompt medical attention.

IX. POISONING BY INSECTS

A. Kinds and effects

1. Stings from ants, bees, wasps, hornets, and yellow jackets occasionally cause death. Death from the sting of such creatures is almost always due to acute allergic reaction.

2. Bites or stings from fleas, mosquitoes, lice, gnats, chiggers, and other common insects produce local pain and irritation but are not likely to cause severe reactions. Some of these insects may transmit disease to man but are not harmful in themselves.

3. Ticks (Fig. 46) can transmit germs of several diseases, including Rocky Mountain spotted fever, a disease that occurs in the eastern portion of the United States as well as the western portion. Ticks adhere tenaciously to the skin or scalp. There is some evidence that the longer an infected tick remains attached, the greater is the chance that it will transmit disease.

4. Spiders in the United States are generally harmless, with two notable exceptions: the black widow spider (Fig. 47)—Latrodectus mactans—and the brown recluse (Loxosceles reclusa) or violin spider (Fig. 48).

a. Symptoms resulting from the black widow spider bite

(1) Slight local reaction

(2) Severe pain produced by nerve toxin

(3) Profuse sweating

(4) Nausea

(5) Painful cramps of abdominal muscles

(6) Difficulty in breathing and speaking

(Victims in almost all cases recover, but an occasional death is reported.)

b. Symptoms resulting from the brown recluse spider bite:

    (1) Severe local reaction, produced by venom, which forms an open ulcer within from 1 to 2 weeks

    (2) Destruction of red cells and other blood changes

    (3) Development of chills, fever, joint pains, nausea and vomiting

    (4) Possible development of generalized rash within from 24 to 48 hours

5. Tarantulas (Fig. 49), identified as hairy spiders, do not ordinarily produce generalized reactions but may be responsible for a severe local wound. They are commonly found in bananas and fruit shipped from South and Central America.

6. Scorpions

Scorpions (Fig. 50) inject venom through a stinger in the tail.

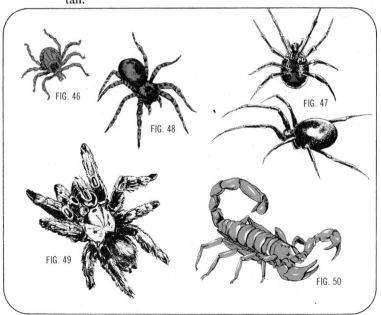

FIG. 46

FIG. 48

FIG. 47

FIG. 49

FIG. 50

a. Effects

In bites from the more dangerous species, there are marked systemic effects within from 1 to 2 hours. Fatalities have been recorded.

b. Symptoms

    (1) Excruciating pain at the site of the sting

    (2) Nausea and vomiting

    (3) Abdominal pain

    (4) Shock

    (5) Possible development of convulsions and coma

B. <u>First aid</u>

  1. Minor bites and stings

    a. Cold applications

    b. Soothing lotions, such as calamine

  2. Tick bites

    a. Cover the tick with heavy oil (mineral, salad, or machine) to close its breathing pores. The tick may disengage at once; if not, allow the oil to remain in place for a half hour. Then carefully remove the tick with tweezers, taking care that all parts are removed.

    b. With soap and water, thoroughly but gently scrub the area from which the tick has been removed, because disease germs may be present on the skin. (Although use of tweezers for removal of a tick and application of heat to the tick's body, as by a lighted cigarette, often have been attempted, these methods may leave tick parts in the wound or may injure the skin.)

3. Severe reactions

a. Give artificial respiration if indicated.

b. Apply a constricting band above the injection site on the victim's arm or leg (between the site and the heart). Do not apply tightly. You should be able to slip your index finger under the band when it is in place.

c. Keep the affected part down, below the level of the victim's heart.

d. If medical care is readily available, leave the band in place; otherwise, remove it after 30 minutes.

e. Apply ice contained in a towel or plastic bag, or cold cloths, to the site of the sting or bite.

f. Give home medicine, such as aspirin, for pain.

g. If the victim has a history of allergic reactions to insect bites or is subject to attacks of hay fever or asthma, or if he is not promptly relieved of symptoms, call a physician or take the victim immediately to the nearest location where medical treatment is available. In a highly sensitive person, do not wait for symptoms to appear, since delay can be fatal.

h. In case of a bee sting, remove and discard the stinging apparatus and venom sac.

X. POISONING BY VENOMOUS SNAKES

A. Kinds and effects

1. Kinds

a. Rattlesnakes—13 species (Fig. 51)

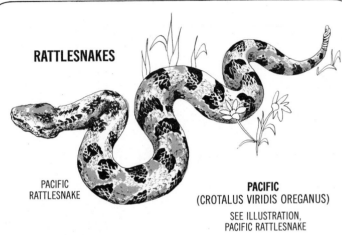

RATTLESNAKES

PACIFIC
RATTLESNAKE

TIMBER
(CROTALUS HORRIDUS)
ALSO CALLED:
**BANDED RATTLESNAKE, MOUNTAIN
RATTLER, AND BLACK RATTLER**
FOUND: In uplands and mountains from
southern Maine to northern Florida and
westward to central Texas.
SIZE: Up to 6 feet; average 4 feet.

DIAMONDBACK
(CROTALUS ADAMANTEUS)
FOUND: From central coast region of
North Carolina; along lower coastal
plain through Florida; westward to
eastern Louisiana.
SIZE: Up to 8 feet.

PACIFIC
(CROTALUS VIRIDIS OREGANUS)
SEE ILLUSTRATION,
PACIFIC RATTLESNAKE
FOUND: British Columbia to southern
California and lower California;
east to Idaho, Nevada, and Arizona.
SIZE: Up to 5 feet.

MASSASAUGA
(SISTRURUS CATENATUS)
ALSO CALLED:
PIGMY RATTLESNAKE
FOUND: Western New York and north-
western Pennsylvania; westward to
northeastern Kansas on the south and
southeastern Minnesota on the north.
A subspecies extends into Texas,
Arizona, and Colorado.
SIZE: Up to 3 feet.

FIG. 51

b. Copperheads (Fig. 52)

c. Cottonmouth moccasins (Fig. 53)

d. Coral snakes (Fig. 54)

COPPERHEAD
(AGKISTRODON MOKESON)
ALSO CALLED:
HIGHLAND MOCCASIN, RATTLESNAKE PILOT, COPPERSNAKE, AND CHUNKHEAD

FOUND: Massachusetts to northern Florida; westward to Mississippi River in Illinois and across to Texas. Found in hilly, rocky country and in lowlands; in walls, hedges, slab sawdust piles, haystacks, barns, and even in villages and towns.
SIZE: Up to 53 inches; average 3 feet.

FIG. 52

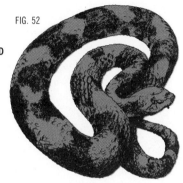

WATER MOCCASIN
(AGKISTRODON PISCIVORUS)
ALSO CALLED:
COTTONMOUTH AND WATER PILOT

FOUND: From southeastern Virginia, along coastal plains through Florida, westward to Texas, and up the Mississippi Valley to Indiana.
SIZE: Up to 39 inches.

FIG. 53

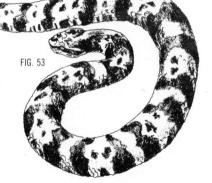

CORAL SNAKE
(MICRURUS FULVIUS)
ALSO CALLED:
HARLEQUIN AND BEAD SNAKE

FOUND: Along the coastal plains from central North Carolina, through Florida, westward to Texas, and up the Mississippi Valley to Indiana.
SIZE: Up to 39 inches.

FIG. 54

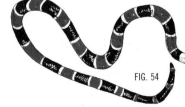

Rattlesnakes, copperheads, and cottonmouth moccasins belong to the family of pit vipers (Crotalidae). These snakes have a pit between the eye and the nostril on each side of the head, elliptical pupils, two well-developed fangs, and one row of plates beneath the tail. Venom of these snakes affects the circulatory system.

The coral snake is a variety of cobra, found along the coast and lowlands of the southeastern United States and in the southwestern portions. The coral snake is small; has tubular fangs, with teeth behind the fangs. It has some features of nonpoisonous snakes: round pupils and a double row of plates beneath the tail. It is characterized by having red, yellow, and black rings around the body, with the red and yellow adjoining, and always has a black nose. The potent venom of the coral snake affects the nervous system and is very toxic.

Nonpoisonous snakes have round pupils, no fangs or pits, and a double row of plates beneath the tail.

All reactions from snakebite are aggravated by acute fear and anxiety.

2. Effects

Factors that affect the severity of local and general reaction from poisonous snakebite include the following:

a. The amount of venom injected and the speed of absorption of venom into the victim's circulation.

b. The size of the victim.

c. Protection from clothing, including shoes and gloves.

d. Specific antivenin therapy, as soon as possible.

e. Location of the bite.

B. Signs and symptoms

1. Pit viper bite

a. Characteristics

(1) Extremely painful.

(2) Characterized by rapid swelling.

(3) Identified by one or more puncture wounds created by the fangs (Fig. 55).

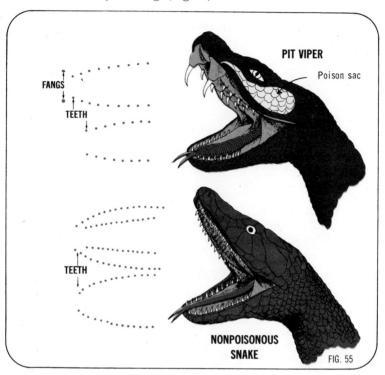

FANGS

TEETH

PIT VIPER

Poison sac

TEETH

NONPOISONOUS
SNAKE

FIG. 55

(4) Usually marked with general discoloration of the skin.

b. Manifestations

General weakness, rapid pulse, nausea and vomiting, shortness of breath, dimness of vision and shock.

2. Coral snake bite – manifestations

Only slight burning pain and mild local swelling at the wound; blurring vision, drooping eyelids, slurring speech, drowsiness, increased saliva and sweating, perhaps nausea and vomiting, shock, respiratory difficulty, paralysis, convulsions, and possible development of coma.

C. Objectives of first aid

   1. To reduce the circulation of blood through the bite area

   2. To delay absorption of venom

   3. To prevent aggravation of the local wound and to sustain respiration

D. <u>First aid</u> procedure

Keep the victim quiet and reassure him. Transport the victim to a source of medical assistance as quickly as possible.

   1. Immobilize the arm or leg in a lowered position, keeping the involved area *below* the level of the victim's heart.

   2. If the bite is on an arm or leg, apply a constricting band from 2 to 4 inches above the bite, between the wound and the victim's heart (Fig. 56). The constricting band should *not* be tight; if it is properly adjusted, there will be some oozing from the wound. You should be able to slip your index finger under the band when it is in place.

   3. Use the blade in a snakebite kit, if available; otherwise, sterilize a knife blade with a flame, and make incisions through the skin at each fang mark and over the suspected venom deposit point. (The snake strikes downward, and the deposit point will be lower than the fang marks.) Be very careful to make the incisions through the skin only and in the long axis of the limb. Do *not* make cross-cut incisions. The incisions must not be deeper than the skin because of the danger of severing muscles and nerves. Special care is necessary in making incisions on the hand, wrist, or foot, because muscles, nerves, and tendons lie close to the surface, and the injury may cause

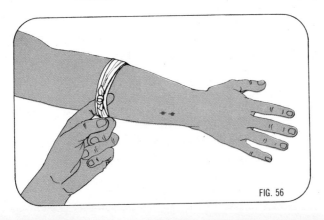

FIG. 56

considerable disability. Do not make incisions more than one-half inch long.

4. Apply suction with the suction cup contained in the snakebite kit, if available; otherwise, use your mouth. Snake venom is not a stomach poison but it should not be swallowed, and you should rinse it from your mouth. Continue suction for from 30 to 60 minutes. If swelling extends up to the constricting band, apply another band a few inches above the first, but leave the first band in place.

5. Wash the wound thoroughly with soap and water and blot dry. Apply a sterile or clean dressing and bandage it in place.

6. You may place a cold, wet cloth or ice wrapped in a cloth, if available, over the wound to slow absorption but do not pack the wound in ice.

7. *Do not* give alcohol in any form.

8. Treat the victim for shock. Unless nausea and vomiting develop, sips of fluid may be given if the victim is conscious and can swallow without difficulty.

9. Give artificial respiration if indicated.

10. Consult a physician with regard to antibiotic therapy and prevention of tetanus, even if the bite has been inflicted by a nonpoisonous snake.

11. If the victim must walk, make sure that he moves slowly.

12. Telephone ahead to the nearest hospital or doctor so that antivenin can be made available quickly.

XI. PREVENTION OF ACCIDENTAL POISONING

Accidental poisoning is a common cause of sudden illness, particularly with children. While most such accidental illnesses do not result in fatality, the death rate from poisoning is serious enough to require every possible prevention effort. Effective prevention is essentially a matter of recognizing the toxic properties of the many products that actually are poisonous and taking necessary protective measures to eliminate the possibility of known poisons entering the body.

A. Swallowed poisons

Most accidental poisonings are the result of swallowing liquid or solid toxic substances. Drugs and chemicals present the most serious hazard. Aspirin, barbiturates, and tranquilizers can be found in many homes, often in exceedingly large quantities. The toxic effects of chemicals in cosmetics, laundry and cleaning products, insecticides, pesticides, and paints or thinners are seldom understood and frequently ignored. If these substances are accessible to unsuspecting hands, they present a serious poisoning hazard.

While the elimination of all poisonous substances commonly found in the home is obviously impractical, the danger of poisonous substances must be recognized, and measures must be taken that will afford maximum protection to oneself and others. Accidental poisoning from drugs and chemicals would be virtually eliminated in the home environment if people would merely read and heed the directions and warnings on container labels and control the accessibility of these items so that young children could not get to them.

All drugs and medicines are potentially poisonous when not taken according to a doctor's instructions or the instructions on the container label. An overdose can interfere with the normal function of one or several of the body's systems and produce a reaction that may range in severity from dulling of the senses to death. If a manufactured household product presents a poison hazard, a warning or caution about this hazard is usually printed on the container. The ease or simplicity of use, as often demonstrated by advertisements of the product, is no excuse for failure to read and heed such warnings.

Perhaps the most dangerous poison-producing condition in the home is the accessibility of the container and its content to an uninformed, unsuspecting person. Danger of accidental handling and swallowing is particularly apt to occur with young children. Container, chemical, and pharmaceutical manufacturers are in constant search for safety design features that will prevent or discourage the opening of bottles and other drug or chemical containers by unsuspecting young children. Control of content accessibility in containers that harbor poisonous substances is an important aspect of poison prevention.

When adequate safeguards do not exist for controlling accessibility to the content of a container of a poison, then accessibility of the container itself must be controlled. If there are members of a household who are ignorant of the harmful effects of any poisonous substance, and accessibility to the content of a container cannot be absolutely controlled, there is no preventive alternative but to store these items under lock and to keep them locked up except during the very moment when they are being used.

It is equally important that poisonous substances are not transferred from their original container to another container, such as a cup or bowl, and then left in the second container. This type of careless action occurs frequently with laundry and cleaning products and presents a dangerous hazard to young children or unsuspecting adults.

Swallowing of poisons is more common in the home but it also contributes to the accident problem in one's pursuit of outdoor leisure-time activities. Common sources of accidental poisoning in the outdoor environment include plant leaves; fungi that look like mushrooms, berries, and other food; chemicals; or other toxic substances. An adult can and should learn to recognize such hazards; children too young to understand these dangers must be protected.

B. Inhaled poisons

Aside from the more common gas poisoning discussed in the chapter on respiratory emergencies and artificial respiration, there are various poisonous sprays and vapors that contaminate the air we breathe. Glues or resins used to build plastic models, sprayed paints, pesticides, weed killers, and hair sprays are a few such items.

Hazards created by toxic fumes, sprays, and vapors often can be avoided if ample ventilation is provided. In some cases, the danger may be great enough to require that sprays or fume-producing resins be used out of doors.

Manufactured products that present a toxic inhalation problem are labeled with warnings and instructions for controlling the hazards involved. Many such products require the use of protective masks in order to give protection against poisoning. Read container warnings and protective instructions carefully, and follow the advice offered right down to the small print. Remember, accessibility to both the content and the container must also be controlled in the case of these items.

C. Contacted poisons

Many manufactured products that present a toxic inhalation hazard also create the danger of poisoning by absorption through skin tissue. Container warnings and instructions indicate such dangers, as well as what preventive measures should be taken.

A frequent source of skin poisoning is that presented by irritating plants. The most common toxic plants encountered are those of the genus Rhus, such as poison ivy. In addition to being transmitted by direct contact between plant and skin, the toxic extract of poisonous plants can also be transmitted by pets and by the soot produced when these plants are burned.

In confined outdoor areas such as yards or play areas, the poison-producing condition can be eliminated by the use of weed killers or by digging up and disposing of toxic plants. In open spaces, protective clothing and the ability to recognize such plants offer the best opportunity to avoid skin contact. It is possible that desensitization of a person can afford some control over the effects of skin contact with poisonous plants. A person with known sensitivity should consult his physician about such possibilities.

D. Injected poisons

Venom injected beneath the skin surface by stinging or biting insects, poisonous snakes, and certain marine life can produce a severe local reaction at the point of injection, an acute systemic reaction, and, occasionally, death.

Preventive efforts must be directed toward learning the habitat and identity of poisonous insects, snakes, and marine life; avoiding their presence, when possible; and exercising whatever control measures may be available for protective purposes.

Insecticides and repellents help to reduce or control the hazards regarding insect poisoning. In snake-infested areas, protective boots and caution about where one steps or reaches with his hands provide a measure of protection. When swimming or sport diving in waters known or suspected to harbor poisonous marine life, avoid contact with any unknown plant or creature. Poisonous sea creatures usually bite or sting only as a defensive measure.

E. Specific prevention of poisoning from drugs and chemicals

   1. Storage

      a. Store all household chemical products and medicines out of reach and sight of children, preferably in a locked cabinet or closet.

      b. Do not store medicines and chemicals on shelves with food.

      c. Make sure that all medicines are properly labeled.

      d. Keep medicines, chemicals, and cosmetic preparations in their original containers; do not transfer contents to unlabeled bottles, glasses, or cups.

      e. Do not reuse containers that have held potentially harmful substances.

   2. Use

      a. Read labels before taking medicines.

      b. Do not take or give medicine at night without turning on the light.

      c. Protect your skin and eyes when using insect poisons, weed killers, solvents, strong detergents, and cleaning agents.

      d. Use liquids and sprays only in well-ventilated places.

      e. Wear a mask over your mouth and nose when spraying paints, pesticides, and similar preparations.

      f. Do not use gasoline or kerosene for starting fires or for cleaning purposes.

      g. Wash thoroughly after using strong chemicals and remove contaminated clothing at once.

      h. Clean up any spilled liquid.

      i. Avoid taking medicine in the presence of small children.

      j. Safeguard with special precautions all drugs that are colored, flavored, or coated with sugar (including aspirin-containing chewing gum).

    k. Warn small children not to eat or drink medicines, or anything else they may find, without your permission.

    l. Teach children about the danger of alcohol, drugs, and poisonous chemicals.

    m. Do not allow children who are building plastic models to inhale plastic glues or resins for a prolonged period of time.

3. Disposal

    a. Take an inventory of drugs and chemicals in the home.

    b. Discard old drugs periodically, particularly those left over from treatment of special illnesses. Flush the drugs down the drain. Rinse containers and throw them away.

F. Preparation for emergencies

1. Learn what to do in case of overdose of medication or accidental poisoning.

2. Keep first aid supplies on hand and available at all times, as well as the telephone numbers of your physician, hospital, and poison control information center and the police and fire departments.

G. Prevention of poisoning from plants

1. Ingested poisons

    a. Bear in mind that prevention of poisoning in small children depends upon early training *not* to chew on leaves or plants, and not to eat berries that they may find unless they have permission to eat them.

    b. Learn which plants are likely to produce poisoning if swallowed accidentally or if included, by chance, with edible vegetables and berries.

2. Contact with poisonous plants

    a. Learn to identify the poisonous plants in locations where you live and visit.

    b. Make sure that persons with known sensitivity avoid contact with poisonous plants, or consult their physicians regarding desensitization injections.

c. Since poisonous plants are often not recognized as such or are identified only after contact, make sure that all persons who have been handling wildflowers, leaves, and plants remove contaminated clothing and thoroughly wash exposed surfaces of the skin as soon as possible.

d. If irritating plants are being burned, stay away, because the soot may contain active substances that produce reaction. The toxic extract of poisonous plants may also be transmitted by pets and on clothing.

8

DRUGS AND THEIR ABUSE

Administered under medical direction, drugs often appear to have miraculous effect in relieving suffering, combating disease, and saving life. When the same drugs are misused or abused, they can become enemies.

I. DEFINITIONS

A. Drug

A drug is a substance that affects the functions of the body or mind when taken into the body or applied to its surface. Some drugs are readily available and are sold over the counter as home remedies. Most drugs, however, are subject to some control or regulation for the protection of health and the promotion of well-being. These drugs are available only on a physician's prescription and are intended to be administered only under the direction of the physician. Such use of drugs constitutes accepted medical practice.

Note that the word *drug* is defined broadly here and is not synonymous with the word *medicament*. Abuse of some substances that are not used in medical practice but are drugs by definition may be particularly widespread and hazardous.

B. Drug misuse

Drug misuse is the use of drugs for purposes or conditions for which they are unsuited or for appropriate purposes but in improper dosage.

C. Drug abuse

Drug abuse is the excessive or persistent use of a drug without regard to accepted medical practice.

D. Drug dependence

Drug dependence is the condition that results from drug abuse. It is described as the interaction between the drug and the body when this interaction involves an effect on the central nervous system. It is characterized by a behavioral response that always includes a compulsive desire to continue taking the drug, either to experience its effects or to avoid the discomfort of its absence. Dependence always involves psychic craving (psychic dependence) and sometimes involves physical, organic disturbance (physical dependence).

II. IDENTIFICATION OF DRUG ABUSE

Almost any drug can be misused or abused. Some drugs are commonly abused, constituting personal and public health problems, with social, economic, and legal implications.

In cases of drug abuse emergency, it is important that the signs and symptoms of the abuse are identified by the person providing the immediate assistance. The type and amount of substance used and the time it was taken should be determined, if possible. When the drugs have been taken by mouth and if the individual is seen at the time of oral ingestion or within a few minutes afterward, an effort to empty the stomach to prevent absorption is recommended.

It is sometimes difficult to distinguish between types of drugs taken merely by observing symptoms. This difficulty is increased when drugs are used in combination. The necessary clues to identification are often provided by apparatus, such as teaspoons, paper packs, eye-droppers, hypodermic needles, vials, or collapsible tubes. The presence of gelatin capsules, pills, or other drug containers, or of needle marks (Fig. 57) on a victim's body is also significant and should be noted.

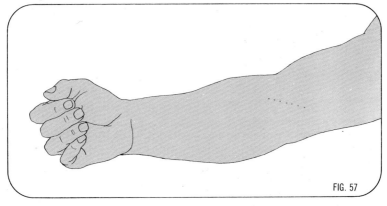

FIG. 57

Information on the types of drugs taken, plus information on the age and size of the victim and his general condition and behavior, should be provided to the drug abuse center or the attending physician.

III. CLASSIFICATION OF DRUGS

Drugs that are abused can be classified in many ways. Some of the groups overlap in one or more effect. The following list is arranged for convenience, without regard to importance, severity, or prevalence of abuse:

- Alcohol (alcoholic beverages)
- Cannabis (marihuana)
- Depressants (sedatives-hypnotics)
- Hallucinogens
- Inhalants
- Narcotics
- Stimulants
- Tranquilizers

A. Alcohol

In this context, the term *alcohol* refers to alcoholic beverages, whose effects relate to their alcoholic content and to the level of alcohol in the blood resulting from their use. The use of alcohol is legal and widely accepted socially in the United States and in many other countries. In spite of this acceptance, prolonged abuse and consumption of large amounts of alcohol may cause great social and economic detriment, as well as physical damage to individual users.

Even a moderate amount of alcohol in combination with a barbiturate or minor tranquilizer may be hazardous.

1. Effects

Alcohol is a depressant, affecting first the higher reasoning areas of the brain, with perhaps a feeling of relaxation or, in the company of others, a sense of exhilaration and conviviality due to the release of inhibitions. Later, motor activity, motor skills, and coordination are disrupted and, with deepening intoxication, other bodily processes are

disturbed. In the most severe stages of alcoholic intoxication, superficial blood vessels are dilated, causing a feeling
of warmth, even though the actual effect is an increased
loss of body heat. Respiration decreases, consciousness
wanes, and coma or death may result.

2. Abuse

The drinker may use alcohol as a psychological "crutch."
Thus, he may develop a psychic, and later a physical,
dependence similar to that produced by the barbiturates.

There is a well-defined alcohol abstinence syndrome
closely related to that described for the barbiturates. De-
lirium tremens is a major symptom complex of alcohol
withdrawal.

The odor of alcohol on a person's breath does not neces-
sarily indicate intoxication. In addition to the noting of
information on incoordination, disturbance of speech, and
altered respiration, other means are commonly used to
determine whether the level of alcohol in the body equals
or exceeds that of legally defined intoxication.

The drinker is often unaware of detriment to his normal
skills and should be restrained from activity requiring such
skills, particularly driving.

3. First aid

Alcohol intoxication, whether due to an acute overdose or
to prolonged abuse, is treated as follows:

a. If the person is sleeping quietly, his face is of normal
   color, his breathing is normal, and his pulse is regular,
   no immediate first aid is necessary.

b. If the person shows such signs of shock as cold and
   clammy skin, rapid and thready pulse, and abnormal
   breathing, or if he does not respond at all, obtain
   medical aid immediately.

c. Maintain an open airway, give artificial respiration if
   indicated, and maintain body heat.

d. If the victim is unconscious, place him in the coma
position (Fig. 58) so that secretions may drool from his
mouth. This position will usually allow for good respiration.

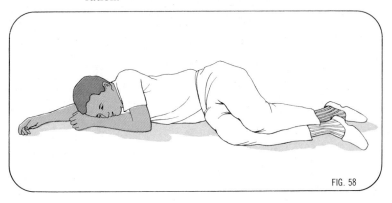

FIG. 58

e. Remember that an intoxicated person may be violent
and obstreperous and will need careful handling to
prevent him from harming himself and others.

The alcoholic should be encouraged to seek help from
Alcoholics Anonymous or from a drug abuse treatment
center.

B. Cannabis (marihuana)

Cannabis sativa is an herbaceous annual plant that grows
wild in temperate climates in many parts of the world. The
various forms of the drug are frequently referred to as cannabis, although the official definition states that cannabis is "the
flowering or fruiting tops of the cannabis plant from which
the resin has not been extracted." Marihuana usually consists
of crushed cannabis leaves and flowers, and often twigs. It
varies greatly in the content of active material. Hashish is a
preparation of cannabis resin, which is squeezed or scraped
from the plant top and is generally five or more times as
potent as marihuana. Marihuana is smoked; hashish may be
smoked but is also commonly made into a confection or
beverage.

1. Effects

The use of cannabis in medical practice is not presently
recognized. The effects to be described, therefore, are

those experienced in abuse. These effects are dose-related; that is, the effects are dependent upon the content of active material—tetrahydro-cannabinols, in particular. The impression that marihuana is a harmless drug has been fostered by the low content of active material in American samples; however, use of the more potent hashish is increasing. The immediate physical effects of smoking one or more marihuana cigarettes include—

a. Throat irritation

b. Increased heart rate

c. Reddening of the eyes

d. Occasional dizziness, incoordination, or sleepiness

e. Increased appetite

The psychological effects vary from individual to individual and with the amount of the drug taken. Among the effects described are feelings of exhilaration, hilarity, and conviviality, but there is also distortion of time and space perception, and there may be disturbance of psychomotor activity, which would impair driving and other skills.

In some individuals and in connection with excessive use of the drug, a psychotoxic reaction resembling a "bad trip" on LSD may occur.

Many persons try marihuana once or twice and then abandon it; some use it intermittently—usually in the company of others—and many use the drug continually. Marihuana can produce psychic dependence, but there is no evidence of physical dependence, and no withdrawal symptoms follow discontinuance.

2. First aid

There is no need for emergency treatment unless a psychotoxic reaction develops, in which case the approach is the same as that for an LSD "bad trip."

C. Depressants (sedatives-hypnotics)

1. Characteristics and types.

Depressants (downers) are drugs that act on the nervous system, promoting relaxation and sleep. Chief among these drugs are the barbiturates, the more important of which are—

a. Phenobarbital (goofballs)

b. Pentobarbital (yellow jackets)

c. Amobarbital (blue devils)

d. Secobarbital (red devils)

Closely related are the nonbarbiturate sedatives, some of which are—

a. Glutethimide (Doridan)

b. Chloral hydrate (knockout drops)

c. Paraldehyde

2. Effects

A usual therapeutic dose of a barbiturate does not relieve pain but has a calming, relaxing effect that promotes sleep. Reactions include—

a. Relief of anxiety and excitement

b. Tendency to reduce mental and physical activity

c. Slight decrease in breathing

Barbiturates are used to reduce the frequency of convulsions in epileptics, and one in particular—Pentothal—is given intravenously as a preoperative sedative.

An overdose of barbiturates produces unconsciousness, deepening to a coma, from which the victim cannot be roused. Barbiturates are frequently involved in instances of accidental death or intentional suicide.

Some accidental poisonings occur when a person becomes confused, as a dose of barbiturates starts to take effect, and inadvertently takes a second dose. Another cause of accidental poisoning is the mutual enhancement of effect that takes place when a barbiturate is taken in conjunction with alcohol. This combination can be lethal, even in small amounts.

3. Abuse

Barbiturates are commonly abused in two ways:

a. The barbiturate is taken in increasing amounts by persons who have developed tolerance to the drug, and thus require larger and larger doses to feel the desired effects.

b. For a thrill, the barbiturate is injected as an alternate to other drugs that are being abused, particularly amphetamines. Barbiturates can produce dependence, both psychic and physical.

Abrupt discontinuance of barbiturate administration to the dependent person causes the following characteristic withdrawal symptoms:

a. Restlessness, insomnia, and tremors

b. Muscular twitching

c. Nausea and vomiting

d. Convulsions

e. Delusions and hallucinations

The convulsions and the psychotic symptoms seldom occur at the same time. The convulsions are likely to occur on the second or third day of withdrawal, the delusions and hallucinations a little later. The other symptoms usually occur within 24 hours of withdrawal. If the individual is not treated, the symptoms last about a week. Abrupt withdrawal of barbiturates is dangerous. Withdrawal should take place gradually and under medical supervision. The dependent person should be persuaded to get help from a physician or a drug abuse treatment center.

4. First aid

a. Maintain an open airway and give the victim artificial respiration, if indicated.

b. Maintain body temperature.

c. Get the victim to a physician or hospital as soon as possible.

D. Hallucinogens

1. Characteristics and types

Hallucinogens are drugs that are capable of producing mood changes, frequently of a bizarre character; disturbances of sensation, thought, emotion, and self-awareness; alteration of time and space perception; and both illusions and delusions. The most important hallucinogen is lysergic acid diethylamide (LSD). Some others are—

a. Mescaline

b. Psilocybin

c. Morning glory seeds

d. A number of synthetic substances

Since none of these substances presently has been accepted for medical use, the effects to be described are those experienced in abuse.

2. Effects

Abuse of hallucinogens is of the spree type: The drug is taken intermittently, although perhaps as often as several times a week. Many persons develop a psychic drive for repetition of the experience, but physical dependence does not develop. The effects may often seem pleasurable and rewarding but they may also be very unpleasant (a "bad trip"), even in the same individual. LSD, for example, is likely to produce these physical effects:

a. Increased activity through its action on the central nervous system

b. Increased heart rate

c. Increased blood pressure

d. Increased body temperature

e. Dilated (enlarged) pupils (Fig. 59)

DILATED PUPIL

NORMAL PUPIL

PINPOINT PUPIL

FIG. 59

f. Flushed face

The psychological effects of hallucinogens, in general, are highly variable and unpredictable. They include an emergence into consciousness of previously suppressed ideas, strong emotional feeling, an impression of astonishingly lucid thought, a feeling of insight and creativity, and an intensification of sensory impressions. Changes in sensation may also be involved (sounds are seen, ordinary things appear beautiful, colors seem to be heard). A feeling of cosmic oneness, profound religious awareness, and a mood of joy and peace also may mark the use of the hallucinogens.

In the bad trip, or "freak-out," there is an intense experience of fear, or nightmarish terror to the point of panic. Other undesirable effects are—

a. Complete loss of emotional control
b. Paranoid delusions
c. Hallucinations
d. Profound depression
e. Tension and anxiety

Disordered social behavior may also occur. Because of the delusions and disordered sensations, the user may think he is immune to harm, or perhaps able to fly, and may suffer severe physical injury. Flashbacks (sensory replays of previous "trips") are associated with the use of hallucinogenic drugs, such as LSD, and such flashbacks may occur months after the drug has been taken. They may be severe or simply amount to a feeling of dizziness or a temporary blackout.

3. First aid

A person on a "trip," good or bad, needs careful attention, reassurance, and protection from bodily harm or the results of his antisocial behavior.

a. Talk the person down from his disturbing experience in quiet and safe surroundings.

b. Get the victim to a physician or hospital as soon as possible. Two persons should accompany him if possible.

E. Inhalants

Occasional self-administration of volatile substances such as ether or chloroform in order to experience intoxication is a very old practice.

1. Types

In recent years, inhalation of a wide variety of substances, a practice commonly referred to as glue-sniffing, has become widespread among young people in their early teens. The substances inhaled include—

a. Fast-drying glue or cement (such as model airplane glue)

b. Many paints and lacquers and their thinners and removers

c. Gasoline

d. Kerosene

e. Lighter fluids and dry-cleaning fluid

f. Nail polish and remover

The usual methods of inhaling are to hold a cloth over the nose and mouth with some of the substance on it or to cover the head with a paper or plastic bag containing a quantity of the substance.

2. Effects

The effects resulting from the use of inhalants are those experienced in abuse. Reactions are—

a. Initial excitement resulting from release of inhibitions

b. Irritation of the respiratory passages

c. Unsteadiness

d. Drunkenness, with growing depression that deepens even to unconsciousness

A serious potential danger accompanies waning consciousness in a person who uses a bag over his head for inhaling. Failure to remove the bag may result in suffocation.

Some of the propellants in the aerosols that are inhaled are toxic to the heart and can cause death by alteration in the rhythm of the heartbeat. This situation requires prompt and intensive medical attention. Persistent use of inhalants may cause some psychic dependence and may produce pathological changes in the liver and other organs.

3. First aid

   a. If a person is found with a bag or other apparatus over his head, remove it immediately.

   b. If breathing stops, administer artificial respiration.

   c. Obtain medical assistance immediately.

F. Narcotics

1. Types

"Narcotics" refers, in general, to opium and specifically to—

   a. Preparations of opium, such as paregoric

   b. Substances found in opium (Morphine and codeine)

   c. Substances derived from morphine (heroin, Dilaudid, etc.)

   d. Synthetic (laboratory-made) substances that have morphinelike effects, including meperidine or Demerol, methadone or Dolophine

In late 1970, federal laws governing the control of narcotics appropriately excluded cocaine and marihuana from the narcotics classification. Cocaine is a stimulant that effects the central nervous system, and marihuana is a mood- and sense-altering substance.

2. Effects

A therapeutic dose of a narcotic relieves pain and reaction to pain, calms anxiety, and promotes sleep. Common reactions to morphine, heroin, and other morphinelike agents include—

   a. Reduction in awareness of pain

   b. Quieting of tension and anxiety

   c. Decrease in activity

    d. Promotion of sleep

    e. Decrease in breathing and pulse rate

    f. Reduction of hunger and thirst

Some unpleasant reactions to narcotics include sweating, dizziness, nausea, vomiting, and constipation.

An overdose of a narcotic results in—

    a. Lethargy and increasing reduction in activity and awareness

    b. Sleep, deepening to coma (prolonged unconsciousness)

    c. Increasing depression of breathing to the point of respiratory failure

    d. Profuse sweating

    e. Fall in temperature

    f. Muscle relaxation

    g. Contraction of pupils to pinpoint size (see Fig. 59, page 134)—except with meperidine

3. Abuse

The continued administration of a narcotic produces both psychic and physical dependence. Discontinuing the drug causes the appearance of the characteristic, recognizable withdrawal symptoms within from 6 to 24 hours. The symptoms and signs include—

    a. Nervousness, restlessness, and anxiety

    b. Tears and a running nose

    c. Sweating, hot and cold flashes, and gooseflesh

    d. Yawning

    e. Muscular aches and pains in legs, back, and abdomen

    f. Nausea, vomiting, and diarrhea (uncontrollable and continuous)

    g. Loss of appetite and loss of weight

    h. Dilated (enlarged) pupils (see Fig. 59, page 134)

     i. Increased breathing, blood pressure, and body temperature

     j. Intense craving for the drug (for a "fix")

If withdrawal symptoms are in evidence they may be promptly relieved by a dose of the same drug or of another drug in the same group. There is little the lay person can do for the individual in withdrawal except to reassure him and to persuade him to go to a drug treatment center or a physician. Other problems associated with the abuse of narcotics are infection, resulting from the use of unsterile needles, the possibility of developing hepatitis, and malnutrition and dental caries (decay) due to neglect of dietary and hygienic practices.

4. First aid

     a. Arouse the victim, if possible, by lightly slapping him with a cold, wet towel and try to get him on his feet.

     b. Maintain an open airway and administer artificial respiration if indicated.

     c. Maintain body temperature.

     d. Avoid rough treatment of the victim.

     e. Reassure the victim and seek medical assistance as soon as possible.

G. Stimulants

Stimulants (uppers) are used to increase mental activity and to offset drowsiness and fatigue.

1. Types

The most commonly abused stimulants are—

     a. Amphetamine (Benzedrine—bennies, pep pills)

     b. Dextroamphetamine (Dexedrine—dexies)

     c. Metamphetamine (Methedrine—meth, speed, crystal)

     d. Methylphenidate (Ritalin)

All of these act similarly and will be described as exemplified by amphetamine.

Caffeine and cocaine are included among the stimulants. Caffeine is a constituent of coffee, tea, and other beverages. It may produce a very mild psychic dependence but it does not cause personal or social damage. Cocaine, used medically as a local anesthetic, is a powerful central nervous system stimulant.

2. Effects

A therapeutic dose of amphetamine produces the following effects:

a. Alertness

b. Wakefulness

c. Relief from fatigue

d. A feeling of well-being

Mental and physical performance may increase to some extent. Amphetamine reduces hunger and has been widely used for this purpose, although the effect is not well sustained, and the feelings of alertness and wakefulness wear off. Amphetamine increases blood pressure, breathing rate, and general bodily activity. Tolerance to the effects of amphetamine can develop to a high degree, resulting in a demand for increased doses.

An overdose of amphetamine may produce toxic effects when taken orally, but these effects are more common when amphetamine is taken by intravenous injection. Use of amphetamines as antiobesity agents (diet pills) has limited value, and there is little recognized medical need for these drugs, although they are occasionally used in treating narcolepsy (uncontrollable desire for sleep) or hyperkinetic (overactive) states.

3. Abuse

Amphetamine abuse can produce strong psychic dependence and a pronounced degree of tolerance, but not physical dependence.

Prolonged administration of oral doses for diet or fatigue control, because of the accompanying sense of well-being, frequently leads to abuse when doses are increased in an effort to maintain the effect. This abuse produces a psychic dependence on the drug, but withdrawal should be possible without serious incident.

In recent years, a form of amphetamine abuse involving repeated intravenous injection of the drug (usually Methedrine or Dexedrine) has developed. Called a "speed run," this abuse is accompanied by considerable risk to the user and the people around him. The pattern of abuse begins with several days of repeated injections, which increase in size and frequency. The daily total sometimes reaches more than 100 times the initial dose. At first, the user may feel energetic, talkative, enthusiastic, happy, and confident. He does not sleep and usually eats little or nothing. After a few days, unpleasant symptoms appear and increase as the dosage increases. These symptoms include—

a. Confusion

b. Disorganization

c. Compulsive repetition of small, meaningless acts

d. Irritability

e. Suspiciousness

f. Fear

g. Hallucinations and delusions, which may become paranoid

h. Aggressive and antisocial behavior, which may endanger others

The run, which usually lasts less than a week, is abruptly terminated. The abuser is left exhausted. He sleeps— sometimes for several days—and, upon awakening, is emotionally depressed, lethargic, and extremely hungry. Shortly, another run is begun, and the cycle is repeated. There is little that can be done for the victim except to protect him against injury and to seek psychiatric help for him for his delusions and hallucinations.

Abuse of cocaine may take a form similar to the speed run, with rapid, repeated intravenous injections followed by psychotoxic symptoms similar to those characteristic of amphetamine, particularly delusions of a paranoid nature. Another cocaine abuse practice is the taking of the drug alternately or concurrently with heroin. In combination, cocaine provides the "up" and heroin the "down." Cocaine abuse results in strong psychic dependence but not physical dependence.

4. First aid

   a. Protect the victim against injury.

   b. Maintain an open airway and administer artificial respiration if indicated.

   c. Maintain body temperature.

   d. Obtain psychiatric help for the victim for his delusions and hallucinations.

H. Tranquilizers

1. Types and abuse

   Agents in this category are commonly referred to as major and minor tranquilizers.

   The major tranquilizers include the phenothiazines (chlorpromazine, for example) and reserpine. They are used in treating mental disease to calm psychotic patients. They have not produced dependence, but overdosage of these drugs produces a deepening state of unconsciousness, a fall in body temperature and blood pressure, and eventual respiratory failure. The effects produced by an overdose are prolonged, and the victim must be watched carefully as long as severe central nervous system depression persists.

   The minor tranquilizers are used to calm anxiety and other feelings of stress and excitement without producing sleep. At high dose levels, their effects are virtually indistinguishable from the effects of the sedative-hypnotics. Common examples of minor tranquilizers are—

   a. Meprobamate (Miltown, Equanil)

   b. Chlordiazepoxide (Librium)

   c. Ethchlorvynol (Placidyl)

   d. Diazepam (Valium)

   Some tranquilizers are used in treating chronic alcoholism, but in effect, this usage represents substitution of one depressant drug for another. These drugs are useful in treating acute alcohol withdrawal.

Prolonged administration of a minor tranquilizer, with a tendency to increase the dose, may result in psychic and physical dependence. The characteristics of dependence on minor tranquilizers and the related withdrawal symptoms are similar to those produced by barbiturates.

2. First aid

    a. Arouse the victim, if possible, by lightly slapping him with a cold, wet towel and try to get him on his feet.

    b. Maintain an open airway and administer artificial respiration if indicated.

    c. Maintain body temperature.

    d. Get the victim to a physician, hospital, or drug abuse treatment center as soon as possible.

9

BURNS

I. DEFINITION

A burn is an injury that results from heat, chemical agents, or radiation. It may vary in depth, size, and severity, causing injury to the cells in the affected area.

II. CAUSES AND EFFECTS

 A. Causes

 Burns are caused most commonly by—

 1. Carelessness with matches and in cigarette smoking
 2. Scalds from hot liquids
 3. Defective heating, cooking, and electrical equipment
 4. Use of open fires that produce flame burns, especially when flammable clothing is worn
 5. Unsafe practices in the home, in the use of flammable liquids for starting fires, for cleaning, and for scrubbing wax off floors
 6. Immersion in overheated bath waters
 7. Use of chemicals, such as lye, strong acids, and strong detergents

 B. Hazards

 In addition to surface burns and the effects of heat on the blood and on body tissues other than the skin, the hazards of fire include the following:

1. Inhaling very hot (superheated) air or irritating or poison-ous gases, including carbon monoxide

2. Asphyxia from insufficient oxygen in the air

3. Falls and injuries from collapsing walls in burning build-ings

III. CLASSIFICATION

Burns are usually classified according to depth or degree of skin damage. Often the degree will differ in various parts of the same affected area.

A. First degree

First-degree burns (Fig. 60) are those resulting from overex-

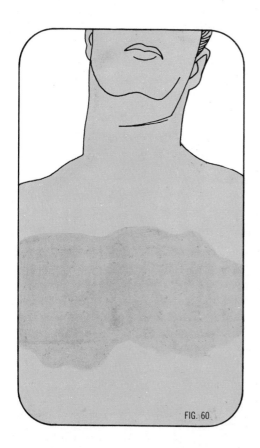

FIG. 60

posure to the sun, light contact with hot objects, or scalding by hot water or steam. The usual signs are—

1. Redness or discoloration

2. Mild swelling and pain

3. Rapid healing

NOTE. Severe sunburn should receive medical care as soon as possible.

B. Second degree

Second-degree burns (Fig. 61) are those resulting from a very deep sunburn, contact with hot liquids, and flash burns from gasoline, kerosene, and other products. Second-degree burns are usually more painful than deeper burns in which the nerve endings in the skin are destroyed.

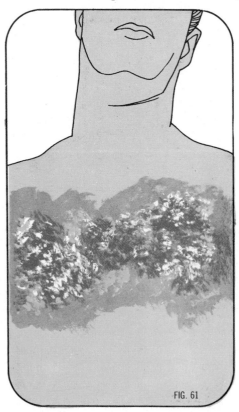

FIG. 61

The usual signs are—

1. Greater depth than first-degree burns

2. Red or mottled appearance

3. Development of blisters

4. Considerable swelling over a period of several days

5. Wet appearance of the surface of the skin, due to the loss of plasma through the damaged layers of the skin

C. Third degree

Third-degree burns (Fig. 62) can be caused by a flame, ignited clothing, immersion in hot water, contact with hot objects, or electricity. Temperature and duration of contact are important factors in determining the extent of tissue destruction.

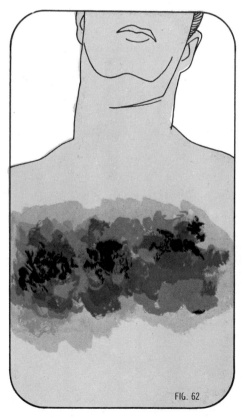

FIG. 62

The usual signs are—

1. Deep tissue destruction

2. White or charred appearance (At first, the burn may resemble a second-degree burn.)

3. Complete loss of all layers of the skin

IV. EXTENT AND LOCATION

In addition to classification of burns according to depth or degree, burns are ordinarily described according to the extent of the total body surface involved.

In general, an adult who has suffered burns of 15 percent of his body surface (a child, 10 percent), wherever located, requires hospitalization. Burns of the face are often associated with injury to the respiratory tract, and may obstruct breathing as swelling increases. Prompt medical attention is imperative.

V. FIRST AID

The objective of first aid for burns is to relieve pain, prevent contamination, and treat for shock. Usually, medical treatment is not required.

A. First-degree burns

1. Apply cold water applications, or submerge the burned area in cold water (Fig. 63).

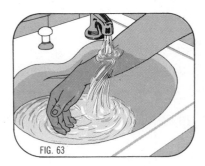

FIG. 63

2. Apply a dry dressing if it is necessary.

B. Second-degree burns

1. Immerse the burned part in cold water (*not* ice water) until the pain subsides.

2. Apply freshly ironed or laundered cloths that have been wrung out in ice water.

3. Blot dry, gently.

4. Apply dry, sterile gauze or clean cloth as a protective bandage.

5. Do not break blisters or remove tissue.

6. Do not use an antiseptic preparation, ointment, spray, or home remedy on a severe burn.

7. If the arms or legs are affected, keep them elevated.

C. Third-degree burns

1. Do not remove adhered particles of charred clothing.

2. Cover burns with thick, sterile dressings or a freshly ironed or laundered sheet or other household linen.

3. If the hands are involved, keep them above the level of the victim's heart.

4. Keep burned feet or legs elevated. (The victim should not be allowed to walk.)

5. Have victims with face burns sit up or prop them up and keep them under continuous observation for breathing difficulty. If respiration problems develop, an open airway must be maintained.

6. Do not immerse an extensive burned area or apply ice water over it, because cold may intensify the shock reaction. However, a cold pack may be applied to the face or to the hands or feet.

7. Arrange transportation to the hospital as quickly as possible.

8. If medical help or trained ambulance personnel will not reach the scene for an hour or more and the victim is *conscious* and *not vomiting*, give him a weak solution of salt and soda at home and en route: 1 level teaspoonful of salt and 1/2 level teaspoonful of baking soda to each quart of water, neither hot nor cold. Allow the victim to sip slowly. Give about 4 ounces (a half glass) to an adult over

a period of 15 minutes. Give about 2 ounces to a child from 1 to 12 years of age, and about 1 ounce to an infant under 1 year of age. Discontinue fluid if vomiting occurs.

If medical help will not be available within an hour or more, fluids may be given if not otherwise contraindicated. (Do not give alcohol.)

9. Do not apply ointment, commercial preparations, grease, or other home remedy. (Such substances may cause further complications and interfere with treatment by the physician.)

D. Chemical burns of the skin

For chemical burns of the skin, first aid steps are—

1. Wash away the chemical with large amounts of water, using a shower or hose, if available, as quickly as possible and for at least 5 minutes. Remove the victim's clothing from the areas involved (Fig. 64).

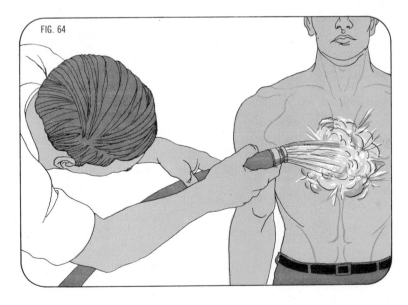

FIG. 64

2. If first aid directions for burns caused by specific chemicals are available, follow these directions after the initial flushing with water.

3. Apply a dressing bandage and get medical aid.

E. Burns of the eye

1. Acid burns

First aid for acid burns of the eye should begin as quickly as possible by thoroughly washing the face, eyelids, and eye for at least 5 minutes. If the victim is lying down, turn his head to the side, hold the eyelids open, and pour water from the inner corner of the eye outward (Figs. 65 and 66). Make sure the chemical does not wash into the other eye.

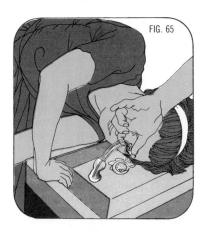
FIG. 65

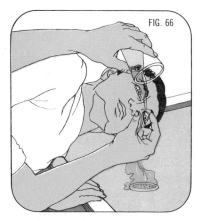
FIG. 66

a. If a weak soda solution (1 teaspoonful of baking soda added to 1 quart of water) can be made quickly, use the solution after first washing the eye with tap water.

b. Cover the eye with a dry, clean, protective dressing (do *not* use cotton) and bandage in place.

c. Caution the victim against rubbing his eye.

d. Get medical help immediately (preferably, an eye specialist).

2. Alkali burns

Alkali burns of the eye can be caused by drain cleaner, strong laundry and dishwater detergents, or other cleaning solutions and are progressive injuries. An eye that first appears to have only slight surface injuries may develop deep inflammation and tissue destruction, and the sight may be lost.

a. First aid

(1) Flood the eye thoroughly with water for 15 minutes.

(2) If the victim is lying down, turn his head to the side. Hold the lids open and pour the water from the inner corner outward.

(3) Remove any loose particles of dry chemicals floating on the eye, by lifting them off gently with a sterile gauze or a clean handkerchief (Fig. 67).

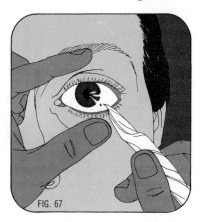

FIG. 67

(4) Do not irrigate with soda solution.

(5) Immobilize the eye by covering it with a dry pad or protective dressing.

(6) Seek immediate medical aid.

3. Irritating gases

a. Effects

Injuries to the eyes from irritating gases are common, and lung damage also may result if sufficient quantity is involved. Many drugs and chemicals are used in spray form. Tear gas in concentrated form may cause blindness and should be handled carefully.

b. First aid

First aid consists of irrigation of the eyes with large quantities of water.

F. Prevention of sunburn

The most effective sunburn prevention lies in limiting the
length of initial exposures at the beginning of warm weather
each year, especially for individuals sensitive to the sun. For
swimming and sunbathing, the first exposure should not be
longer than 15 minutes, with gradual increases of from 5 to
10 minutes. On beaches and while boating or fishing during
the summer, however, both children and adults should avoid
long exposures from midmorning until midafternoon. Sunburn may develop following exposure even on a cloudy day.
Persons engaged in outdoor work or sports should wear protective clothing during this critical period, and those with
light complexions should cover their hands and faces with
suitable ultraviolet-light-screening preparations.

Commercial preparations for sunburn protection vary in their
effects. Most preparations contain oils to keep the skin from
drying on exposure to heat, wind, and water. Some have
hardly any protective effects; others are highly effective but
expensive. Many of these preparations may cause allergic
reactions in individual cases. A small sample should be tested
on the skin before liberal amounts are used. Preparations that
protect against ultraviolet rays should be reapplied after
swimming.

The eyes, as well as the skin, should be protected, either by
shade or by sunglasses, against irritation from overexposure to
the glare of sun, sand, water, ice, and snow.

VI. PREVENTION OF HEAT EMERGENCIES

The following information relates to the more common conditions and activities that produce heat emergencies. A responsible
attitude toward acquiring additional preventive information, particularly in regard to fires and burns, should lead the reader to
resources beyond the basic discussion contained herein.

A. Injuries from extreme heat

Fires, burns, and other emergencies produced by fire are the
third leading cause of accidental death. About 20 percent of
the fatalities are children. The home environment is particularly dangerous. Some four out of five deaths due to fire occur
in the home. In addition, numerous persons are affected by

nonfatal burn injuries each year. Prevention of burns is, essentially, a matter of preventing fires, as well as protection of self and others from sources of extreme heat other than fire.

1. Smoking and matches

Home fires and burn injuries are often the result of children playing with matches and careless handling of matches by adults. When the hazards of dangerous play are not fully understood by children, protective measures similar to those controlling accessibility to dangerous poisons should be followed. Careless handling or disposal of matches and lighted cigarettes is a primary factor in the cause of about 25 percent of all fires of known origin.

Smoking while in bed is one of the most frequent causes of fire in homes and places of public accommodation. In addition to the danger of burns, a fire in bedding also releases toxic gases that can quietly suffocate sleeping persons in the room or in other parts of the building. Considering the number of fire fatalities where smoking in bed has been identified as the primary causative factor, smokers should see that the practice seems most unwise.

2. Cooking and heating equipment

Cooking and heating equipment is a common source of fires and burns. It is very important that equipment be kept clean and in good repair. A qualified person should inspect and clean heating systems and chimneys annually. If repairs are needed, an expert should be called upon.

Flammable liquids create a special handling and storage problem. If a stove uses fuel oil, store surplus quantities outdoors. Do not use highly flammable liquids for household purposes or for lighting a charcoal grill or other fire. Store flammable liquids in safety containers that seal off explosive vapors from the air. Any flame or spark can produce an explosivelike flash fire wherever a concentration of volatile fumes exists. Similar precautions are necessary where gas is used as a fuel. If a pilot light or gas burner blows out, ventilate thoroughly, and then carefully follow the manufacturer's directions in relighting the unit.

Fire and burn prevention also requires that good housekeeping and safe personal practices be followed in the use of cooking and heating equipment. Cooking surfaces should be kept clean from grease. Turn pot handles so that they do not stick out over the edge of a stove; otherwise, children might pull scalding liquids down upon themselves. Keep portable space heaters out of room traffic lanes and turn them off before going to bed. Make sure that curtains cannot blow across cooking surfaces and that loose clothing is not worn around cooking burners. Remember, too, that children need special protection from these and other potentially hazardous fire situations.

3. Fires of electrical origin

   Fires of electrical origin are usually the result of overloaded or defective wiring, and worn-out or damaged power tools, appliances, fractional horsepower motors, fixture outlets, and cords.

   Many older homes are not electrically wired to accommodate the number of appliances and amount of electrical equipment that are in common use today. In such homes, it is most important that fuses are the right size so that circuits are protected from becoming overloaded. A fuse or a circuit breaker, which acts as a safety valve for overloaded circuits, slows or cuts off the current so that wiring will not overheat and create a fire.

   Fire and burn protection also requires worn-out or damaged tools, appliances, cords, and other electrical items to be either discarded or repaired. Repairs should be made by qualified repairmen. Repairs are particularly important where television sets are concerned. Unless a television set is designed specifically for installation in a tightly enclosed space, do not install it where required ventilation will be obstructed; a fire hazard can be created if adequate ventilation is not provided.

   An absence of grounded circuits and electrical appliances or equipment without grounded wiring poses the ever-present danger that a current of electricity can reach and pass through the body. A three-holed wall receptacle *implies* a grounded circuit. A three-pronged plug on an appliance cord or piece of electrical equipment *implies* that the item is wired to afford protection against electric current's reaching the body provided that the item is plugged into a grounded circuit. Whenever a manufacturer recommends that electrical appliances or equipment should be grounded, follow the advice. If both the circuit and the appliance are improperly wired and plugged for grounding, have a competent electrician inspect the circuit wiring, circuit load, and wall receptacle, and request him to ground the piece of equipment or appliance.

B. Radiation burns

The usual source of radiation burns is an overexposure to the ultraviolet rays of the sun during warm weather seasons. Light-complexioned persons are particularly susceptible to burning by the sun's rays. Sunburn can be prevented by controlling the amount of exposure to ultraviolet rays until a suntan has developed, and by avoiding excessive exposure, particularly during the midmorning to midafternoon period, when the amount of ultraviolet radiation is greatest.

The first few exposures at the beginning of an outdoor season should be limited to periods of no more than 15 minutes. Later exposures should be regulated so that a protective suntan can develop gradually. Commercial skin preparations that are made specifically to screen out ultraviolet rays may also be helpful. Some commercial preparations have little protective effects against ultraviolet rays, and any one of them may cause an allergic reaction in individual cases. A person may wish to check with his own physician for advice in selecting a sunburn prevention preparation. For best results when using a particular preparation, follow directions on the container label.

Persons who spend a great deal of time in the hot sun should avoid excessive exposure by wearing protective clothing and using a sunburn preventive preparation on the hands, neck, and face. Remember, too, that cloudy weather does not ensure protection against ultraviolet ray exposure.

The eyes also need protection from long exposure to sunlight and glare. While a cap visor may shield the eyes from sun, sand, water, ice, and snow glare, protection against sunlight and water or surface reflection is best obtained by wearing sunglasses. Seek professional advice about the selection of effective sunglasses.

C. Chemical burns

Prevention of chemical burns would be almost universally accomplished if people would heed the warnings and carefully read and follow instructions printed on the original containers of products. Eye tissue is particularly vulnerable. Special precautions are necessary in the handling and use of sprays, gases, and the many household and garden products containing caustic chemical compounds that can be splashed or rubbed into the eyes.

Make a normal practice of carefully reading the label of *every* spray can, as well as any package containing laundry or dishwashing products, insecticides, pesticides, hair sprays, deodorants, garden and soil products, antiseptics, or medicines. Since these chemicals are also dangerous if swallowed or inhaled, the same preventive measures regarding security and storage as suggested in the chapter on accidental poisoning should be followed.

D. Specific fire or burn prevention

- Install fire extinguishers in danger spots.
- Keep a garden hose near a faucet for use in case of fire.
- Install adequate insulation at all heating surfaces.
- Repair or replace defective or inadequate electrical wiring.
- Perform the required maintenance on heating systems.
- Dispose of trash immediately.
- Use only nonflammable cleaning fluids.
- Hang clothes well away from stoves or fireplaces.
- Place curtains so that they will not blow into flames from any stove, candle, etc.
- Store flammable materials in a safe place.
- Do not overload electrical circuits.
- Supervise children playing near an open fire.
- Store matches in a metal container and out of reach of children.
- Turn pot and pan handles away from the edge of the stove.
- Do not leave tubs of hot water where children can fall into them.
- Do not smoke in bed.
- Do not smoke if you are sleepy.
- Provide adequate ashtrays throughout the house.
- Install home fire detectors.

E. Escape from fire

Every family should have a fire escape plan that includes at least two possible ways to get outdoors from every room in the house. Emergency exit plans should be discussed and practiced until each family member knows exactly what to do. The two most important things to remember in case of fire are, first, to get everybody out of the house, and then to call the fire department.

Escape from fire is more likely to be accomplished safely if certain basic facts are understood. For example, since heated air and carbon monoxide gas tend to rise, persons should stay close to the floor. Any part of the body covered by a thick cloth, particularly if the cloth is wet, will be protected for a time from heat, but not from fumes. It is especially important to protect the hands, face, and respiratory passages. There is actually no satisfactory protection against carbon monoxide, but the lowest concentration of the gas will be found in air near the floor. If clothing catches fire, do not run; roll on the floor or ground. Smother the flaming clothes of another person with a coat or blanket.

When attempting escape, place the palm of your hand against any inside door before opening it. If the door feels hot, either leave by another exit or wait at a window for rescue. Open the window slightly, from the bottom, so that fresh breathing air can be obtained. Hang clothing or a bedsheet from the window to signal rescuers. If a door feels cool to the touch, open it slightly, staying low and behind the door. The next room may contain superheated air, under pressure, that could explode as it expands. Pass your hand across the door opening, and if the air feels cool, it should be safe to enter.

Close doors behind you upon leaving rooms and the house. Fire travels faster when doors and windows are open. After everybody is safely out of the house, call the fire department, giving your name and the address where the fire is located.

F. Prevention of heat illnesses

The extent to which various body systems can adapt to a hot climate or hot working conditions, exposure to alternately high and low temperature extremes, and conditions of high and low humidity is apparently related to an individual's ability to avoid heat illnesses. This systemic adaptation ability varies among individuals.

Drinking adequate amounts of water and increasing the intake of salt are two preventive measures that may help to avoid heat illness, particularly in the case of heat exhaustion and heat cramps. Restriction of activity, good ventilation and movement of air by fans and air conditioning, moderate eating habits, and the wearing of loose and light-colored clothing in hot, sunny weather can help lower the incidence of heat reactions.

Heat stroke is an immediate, life-threatening problem. The cooling of body surfaces, such as the exposed face, neck, and arms, by periodic sponging with cool water is sometimes helpful in preventing the onset of heat stroke. Exposure and activity should be limited where extremely hot climatic and working conditions permit, particularly in the case of young children, elderly persons, and other people known to be susceptible to the effects of extreme heat.

10

FROSTBITE AND COLD EXPOSURE

The extent of injury caused by exposure to abnormally low temperature generally depends on such factors as wind velocity, type and duration of exposure, temperature, and humidity.

Freezing is accelerated by wind and by humidity or a combination of the two factors.

I. FROSTBITE

A. Characteristics

Frostbite results when crystals form, either superficially or deeply in the fluids and underlying soft tissues of the skin. The effects are more severe if the injured area is thawed and then refrozen. Frostbite is the most common injury resulting from exposure to cold elements. Usually, the frozen area is small. The nose, cheeks, ears, fingers, and toes are most commonly affected.

B. Signs and symptoms

Just before frostbite occurs, the affected skin may be slightly flushed. As frostbite develops—

1. The skin changes to white or grayish-yellow in appearance (Fig. 68).

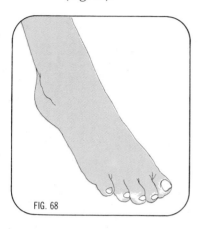

FIG. 68

2. Pain is sometimes felt early but subsides later (often there is no pain).

3. Blisters may appear later.

4. The affected part feels intensely cold and numb.

5. The victim frequently is not aware of frostbite until someone tells him or he observes the *pale, glossy skin.*

As time passes—

1. There is mental confusion and impairment of judgment.

2. The victim staggers.

3. Eyesight fails.

4. The victim falls and may become unconscious.

5. Shock is evident.

6. Breathing may cease.

7. Death, if it occurs, is usually due to heart failure.

C. First aid

1. Objectives

The objectives of first aid are to protect the frozen area from further injury, to warm the affected area rapidly, and to maintain respiration.

2. Procedure

    a. Cover the frozen part.

    b. Provide extra clothing and blankets.

    c. Bring the victim indoors as soon as possible.

    d. Give the victim a warm drink.

    e. Rewarm the frozen part *quickly* by immersing it in water that is warm, but not hot, when tested by pouring some of the water over the inner surface of your forearm. Place a thermometer in the water and carefully add warm water to maintain the temperature between 102° and 105° (Fig. 69). NOTE. If the affected part has

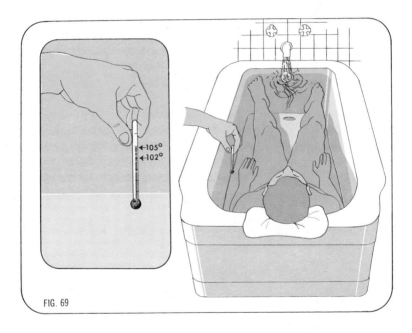

FIG. 69

been thawed and refrozen, it should be warmed at room temperature (from 70°F to 74°F).

    f. If warm water is not available or practical to use, wrap the affected part *gently* in a sheet and warm blankets.

    g. *Do not* rub the part; rubbing may cause gangrene (tissue death).

h. *Do not* apply heat lamp or hot water bottles.

i. *Do not* let the victim bring the affected part near a hot stove.

j. *Do not* break the blisters.

k. *Do not* allow the victim to walk after the affected part thaws, if his feet are involved.

l. Since severe swelling develops very rapidly after thawing, *discontinue* warming the victim as soon as the affected part becomes flushed.

m. Once the affected part is rewarmed, have the victim exercise it.

n. If fingers or toes are involved, place dry, sterile gauze between them to keep them separated.

o. Do not apply other dressings unless the victim is to be transported for medical aid.

p. If travel is necessary, cover the affected parts with sterile or clean cloths and keep the injured parts elevated.

q. Elevate the frostbitten parts and protect them from contact with bedclothes.

r. Give fluids as described in the chapter on burns, provided that the victim is conscious and not vomiting.

s. Obtain medical assistance as soon as possible.

II. COLD EXPOSURE

A. Manifestations

Prolonged exposure to extreme cold produces the following manifestations:

1. Shivering

2. Numbness

3. Low body temperature

4. Drowsiness

5. Marked muscular weakness

B. First aid

1. Give artificial respiration, if necessary.

2. Bring the victim into a warm room as quickly as possible.

3. Remove wet or frozen clothing and anything that is constricting.

4. Rewarm the victim rapidly by wrapping him in warm blankets, or by placing him in a tub of water that is *warm but not hot* to the hand or forearm.

5. If the victim is conscious, give him hot liquids by mouth (not alcohol).

6. Dry the victim thoroughly if water was used to rewarm him.

7. Carry out appropriate procedures as described for frostbite.

III. PREVENTION OF INJURIES FROM EXTREME COLD

Frostbite occurs when skin tissue is subjected to extremely cold atmospheric conditions for a duration of time long enough to result in actual freezing of tissue fluids. Prevention involves limiting, if not avoiding, the duration of exposure to extreme cold, avoiding personal practices that may actually contribute to freezing of tissue, wearing proper protective covering, recognizing early symptoms of the onset of frostbite, and removal from such exposure.

If you must go outdoors into extremely cold air temperatures, particularly if high wind or humidity is also present, limit exposure time as much as possible. The danger of frostbite is increased if you are tired or your body's normal resistance is low because of a recent illness. Do not drink alcoholic beverages, smoke, or bathe immediately prior to going out into extremely cold air. Keep moving about in cold air; exercise fingers and toes if necessary, but avoid overexertion.

The right kind of protective clothing is most important. Thermal-type woolen underclothing; outer garments that will repel wind and moisture; face helmet and head and ear coverings; an extra pair of socks; warm boots; and woolen lined mittens or gloves made of wind- and water-repellent material are all basic items of protective clothing desirable for use in extremely cold weather. Make certain that clothing, particularly footwear, is not so tight that circulation is apt to become restricted. Keep clothing dry.

Finally, learn to recognize the symptoms that indicate possible onset of frostbite. Rest, shelter from wind and moisture, hot drinks, and an opportunity to warm cold body parts or to change damp clothing should be sought quickly when these early symptoms are evidenced. Cold hands may be given some relief by placing them under dry clothing against the body, such as in the armpits.

11

HEAT STROKE, HEAT CRAMPS, AND HEAT EXHAUSTION

Excessive heat may affect the body in a variety of ways, which result in several conditions referred to as heat stroke, heat cramps, and heat exhaustion.

I. DEFINITIONS

A. Heat stroke is a response to heat characterized by extremely high body temperature and disturbance of the sweating mechanism. Heat stroke is an immediate, life-threatening emergency for which medical care is urgently needed.

B. Heat cramps involve muscular pains and spasms due largely to loss of salt from the body in sweating or to inadequate intake of salt. Heat cramps may be associated, also, with heat exhaustion.

C. Heat exhaustion is a response to heat characterized by fatigue, weakness, and collapse due to intake of water inadequate to compensate for loss of fluids through sweating.

II. CAUSES

Heat reactions are brought about by both internal and external factors. Harmful effects occur when the body becomes overheated and cannot eliminate the excess heat. Reactions usually occur when large amounts of water, salt, or both are lost through profuse sweating following strenuous exercise or manual labor in an extremely hot atmosphere. Elderly individuals, small children, chronic invalids, alcoholics, and overweight persons are particularly susceptible to heat reactions, especially during heat waves in areas where a moderate climate usually prevails.

III. HEAT STROKE

A. Signs and symptoms

1. Body temperature is high (may be 106°F or higher).

2. The skin is characteristically hot, red, and dry (Fig. 70). The sweating mechanism is blocked.

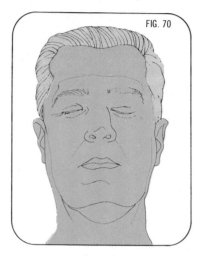

FIG. 70

3. The pulse is rapid and strong.

4. The victim may be unconscious.

B. First aid

First aid should be directed toward *immediate* measures to cool the body quickly. Take care, however, to prevent over-chilling of the victim once his temperature is reduced below 102°F.

The following first aid measures are applicable whenever the body temperature reaches 105°F:

1. Undress the victim and, using a small bath towel to maintain modesty, repeatedly sponge the bare skin with cool water or rubbing alcohol; *or* apply cold packs continuously; *or* place the victim in a tub of cold water (do not add ice) until his temperature is lowered sufficiently. When the victim's temperature has been reduced enough, dry him off.

2. Use fans or air conditioners, if available, because drafts will promote cooling.

3. If the victim's temperature starts to go up again, start the cooling process again.

4. Do not give the victim stimulants.

IV. HEAT CRAMPS

A. Symptoms

In the case of heat cramps, the muscles of the legs and abdomen are likely to be affected first.

B. First aid

1. Exert firm pressure with your hands on the cramped muscles, or gently massage them, to help relieve the spasm.

2. Give the victim sips of salt water (1 teaspoonful of salt per glass), half a glass every 15 minutes, over a period of about 1 hour.

V. HEAT EXHAUSTION

A. Symptoms

1. *Approximately normal* body temperature

2. Pale and clammy skin (Fig. 71)

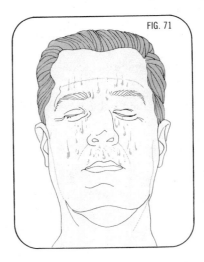

FIG. 71

3. Profuse perspiration

4. Tiredness, weakness

5. Headache—perhaps cramps

6. Nausea—dizziness (possible vomiting)

7. Possible fainting (But the victim will probably regain consciousness as his head is lowered.)

B. First aid

1. Give the victim sips of salt water (1 teaspoonful of salt per glass, half a glass every 15 minutes), over a period of about 1 hour.

2. Have the victim lie down and raise his feet from 8 to 12 inches.

3. Loosen the victim's clothing.

4. Apply cool, wet cloths and fan the victim or remove him to an air-conditioned room.

5. If the victim vomits, do not give him any more fluids. Take the victim as soon as possible to a hospital, where an intravenous salt solution can be given.

6. After an attack of heat exhaustion, advise the victim not to return to work for several days and see that he is protected from exposure to abnormally warm temperatures.

12

SUDDEN ILLNESS

First aid workers often encounter emergencies that are not related to injury but arise from either sudden illness or a crisis in a chronic illness. Unless the illness is minor and brief, such as a fainting attack, airsickness, a nosebleed, or a headache, medical assistance should be sought. Although sudden illness is not always urgent, sometimes it endangers a person's life, especially if associated with a heart attack or a massive internal hemorrhage. An important first aid measure in such an instance is to secure transportation of the victim to receive medical care as quickly and safely as possible.

Many persons suffering from heart disease, apoplexy, epilepsy, or diabetes carry an identification card or bracelet that contains information about the type of illness and the steps to be followed if the persons are found unconscious. Search the victim (in the presence of witnesses) for such identification.

I. HEART ATTACK

Heart attack usually involves a clot in one of the blood vessels that supply the heart. The attack is sometimes called a coronary since there is a loss of blood supply to a portion of the heart muscle (by blockage of the coronary arteries). A heart attack may or may not be accompanied by loss of consciousness. If the attack is severe, the victim may die suddenly. The victim may have a history of heart disease, or the attack may come with little or no warning. Attacks with mild pain sometimes occur. The degree of pain is not a good indication of the seriousness of the disease.

A. Signs and symptoms

    1. Persistent chest pain, usually under the sternum (breast-bone). The pain frequently radiates to one or both shoulders or arms or the neck or jaw or both.

    2. Gasping and shortness of breath

    3. Extreme pallor or bluish discoloration of the lips, skin, and fingernail beds

    4. Extreme prostration

    5. Shock (as a rule)

    6. Swelling of the ankles, which may be an indication of heart disease

The two principal symptoms of an acute heart attack are pain (in the chest, upper abdomen, or down the left arm and shoulder) and extreme shortness of breath. The symptoms can occur together, but usually one or the other is stronger. Indigestion, nausea, and vomiting are often associated with a heart attack.

B. First aid after a heart attack has occurred

    1. Place the victim in a comfortable position, usually sitting up, particularly if there is shortness of breath, although his comfort is a good guide. Use as many pillows as needed.

    2. Provide ventilation and guard against drafts and cold.

    3. If the victim is not breathing, begin artificial respiration.

    4. Have someone call for an ambulance equipped with *oxygen*, and have the victim's own doctor notified.

    5. If the victim has been under medical care, help him with his prescribed medicine. (Look for some form of emergency medical identification.) If in doubt, confer with a physician by telephone.

    6. Do not give liquids to an unconscious victim.

    7. Since transportation throws added strain upon the victim, do *not* attempt to transport him until you get medical advice, if available within a reasonable time.

II. STROKE

A stroke (also called apoplexy) usually involves a spontaneous rupture of a blood vessel in the brain or formation of a clot that interferes with circulation.

A. Major stroke

    1. Signs and symptoms

        a. Unconsciousness

        b. Paralysis or weakness on one side of the body

        c. Difficulty in breathing and in swallowing

        d. Loss of bladder and bowel control

        e. Pupils of the eyes unequal in size

        f. Lack of ability to talk or slurring of speech

    2. First aid

        a. Provide moderate covering.

        b. Maintain an open airway.

        c. Give artificial respiration if indicated.

        d. Position the victim on his side so that secretions will drain from the side of the mouth.

        e. Call a doctor for medical advice as quickly as possible.

        f. *Do not* give fluids unless the victim is fully conscious and able to swallow and unless medical care will be delayed a long time.

B. Minor stroke

In a minor stroke, small blood vessels in the brain are involved. These usually do not produce unconsciousness, and the symptoms depend upon the location of the hemorrhage and the amount of brain damage.

    1. Symptoms

        a. The minor stroke may occur during sleep and be accompanied by—

            (1) Headache

(2) Confusion

(3) Slight dizziness; ringing in the ears

(4) Other mild complaints

b. Later, there may be—

(1) Minor difficulties in speech

(2) Memory changes

(3) Weakness in an arm or leg

(4) Some disturbance in the normal pattern of the personality

2. <u>First aid</u>

a. Protect the victim against accident or physical exertion.

b. Suggest medical attention.

III. FAINTING

Fainting is a partial or complete loss of consciousness due to a reduced supply of blood to the brain for a short time. Occasionally, a person collapses suddenly without warning. Recovery of consciousness almost always occurs when the victim falls or is placed in a reclining position, although injury may occur from the fall. To prevent a fainting attack, a person who feels weak and dizzy should lie down or bend over with his head at the level of his knees.

A. Manifestations

Signs and symptoms are usually preceded or accompanied by—

1. Extreme paleness

2. Sweating

3. Coldness of the skin

4. Dizziness

5. Numbness and tingling of the hands and feet

6. Nausea

    7. Possible disturbance of vision

B. <u>First aid</u>

    1. Leave the victim lying down.

    2. Loosen any tight clothing and keep crowds away.

    3. If the victim vomits, roll him onto his side or turn his head to the side and, if necessary, wipe out his mouth with your fingers, preferably wrapped in cloth.

    4. Maintain an open airway.

    5. *Do not* pour water over the victim's face because of the danger of aspiration; instead, bathe his face gently with cool water.

    6. *Do not* give any liquid unless the victim has revived.

    7. Examine the victim to determine whether or not he has suffered injury from falling.

    8. Unless recovery is prompt, seek medical assistance. The victim should be carefully observed afterward because fainting might be a brief episode in the development of a serious underlying illness.

IV. CONVULSION

A convulsion is an attack of unconsciousness usually of violent onset. In an infant or small child, a convulsion may occur at the onset of an acute infectious disease, particularly during a period of high fever or severe gastrointestinal illness. Convulsions that develop later in the course of measles, mumps, and other childhood diseases are more serious and might reflect complications of the central nervous system.

Convulsions associated with head injury or brain disease, such as a tumor, an abscess, or a hemorrhage, often tend to be localized, with rigidity and jerking of groups of muscles instead of the whole body.

A. Signs and symptoms

    1. Rigidity of body muscles, usually lasting from a few seconds to perhaps half a minute, followed by jerking movements. During the period of rigidity, the victim may stop breathing, bite his tongue severely, and lose bladder and bowel control.

    2. Bluish discoloration of the face and lips.

    3. Foaming at the mouth or drooling.

    4. Gradual subsidence.

B. First aid

    1. Prevent victim from hurting himself.

    2. Give artificial respiration, if indicated.

    3. *Do not* place a blunt object between the victim's teeth.

    4. *Do not* restrain him.

    5. *Do not* pour any liquid into his mouth.

    6. *Do not* place a child in a tub of water.

If repeated convulsions occur, call for medical help immediately or take the victim to a hospital.

V. EPILEPSY

A. Characteristics

Epilepsy is a chronic disease, usually of unknown cause, usually characterized by repeated convulsions—"grand mal" seizures. The victim may be able to lie down quickly, or the family may be able to tell that an attack is beginning by the sudden paleness of his face or by his behavior. The usefulness of mouth-to-nose breathing in providing artificial ventilation for victims of grand mal seizure is effective.

Because of the high incidence of expiratory obstruction created by the soft palate, mouth-to-nose ventilation is the only effective way in which victims with such obstruction can be ventilated. The mouth-to-nose technique must be accomplished in such a way that the mouth is left open for exhalation. If the teeth cannot be separated, the lips should be parted to permit passive exhalation. Much research has been carried out on epilepsy in recent years, and excellent preventive treatment is available; for this reason, physicians should determine the type and cause of every episode of convulsion.

A milder form of epilepsy occurs without convulsions. There may be only brief twitching of muscles, "petit mal" seizures, and momentary loss of contact with the surroundings. The victim may be seen staring fixedly at an object or off into the distance. This type of disturbance is less common than that which produces grand mal seizures.

B. <u>First aid</u>

First aid for epilepsy is the same as for other convulsions, with primary effort being made to prevent the victim from hurting himself.

1. Push away nearby objects.

2. *Do not* force a blunt object between the victim's teeth. (If the victim's mouth is open, you might place a soft object such as a rolled handkerchief between his side teeth.)

3. When jerking is over, loosen the clothing around his neck.

4. Keep him lying down.

5. Keep his airway open.

6. Prevent his breathing of vomit into the lungs by turning his head to one side or by having him lie on his stomach.

7. If breathing stops, give artificial respiration.

8. After the seizure, allow the victim to sleep or rest.

9. If convulsions occur again, get medical help.

VI. PREVENTION OF HEART ATTACK AND APOPLEXY

The following measures may help to prevent a heart attack as well as apoplexy:

• Have a checkup every year after the age of 40.

• Control weight.

• Do not exercise strenuously if you are not used to it.

• Get adequate rest.

13

DRESSINGS AND BANDAGES

Techniques of applying dressings and bandages vary according to the extent and location of injuries, the material at hand, and the ability of the first-aider to adapt to an emergency situation. Supplies can be obtained commercially (Fig. 72) for home use, or substitutes

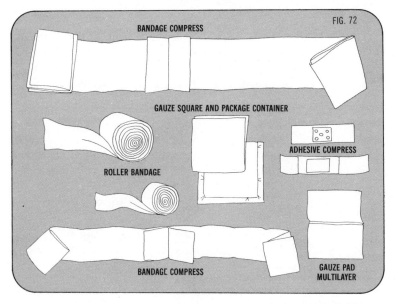

FIG. 72

BANDAGE COMPRESS

GAUZE SQUARE AND PACKAGE CONTAINER

ROLLER BANDAGE

ADHESIVE COMPRESS

BANDAGE COMPRESS

GAUZE PAD MULTILAYER

can be prepared from household linen. It may be necessary to improvise dressings and bandages from any woven fabric available, or even from facial tissues, other paper goods, or unused plastic bags. Fluff cotton, which may be used to pad a splint, should never be placed directly upon an open wound, because the fibers are difficult to remove.

I. DRESSINGS

A. Definition

A dressing, also called compress, is the immediate protective cover placed over a wound. Sterile dressings are those free from germs prior to use and are preferable to unsterile dressings. If sterile dressings are not obtainable, a freshly ironed or laundered cloth, such as a handkerchief, towel, sheet, pillowcase, or napkin may be used.

B. Functions

1. To assist in the control of bleeding

2. To absorb blood and wound secretions

3. To prevent additional contamination

4. To ease pain

C. Sterilizing procedure

To sterilize dressings at home, wrap them in aluminum foil and place them in a moderate oven (350° F) for 3 hours, or boil them for 15 minutes and dry them without contamination. For immediate use, a clean cloth pressed with a hot iron or the inner surface of a folded cloth will usually suffice. Do not touch, or breathe on or cough on the surface of a dressing that is to be placed next to a wound.

Use a dressing large enough to extend an inch or more beyond the edge of the wound. First, hold it over the wound and then lower it into place; do not slide it onto the wound from the side. If a dressing slips off onto surrounding skin before it has been anchored in place, discard it. Secure a dressing with bandages or tape, but *do not* wrap tape completely around the affected part, because blood vessels may be constricted as swelling occurs.

II. BANDAGES

A. Definition

A bandage is a strip of woven material used to hold a wound dressing or splint in place. It helps to immobilize, support, and protect an injured part of the body. Occasionally, large pieces of cloth are used as bandages, as slings, and as binders.

B. Kinds

A bandage must be clean but need not be sterile. The most useful of those available commercially include—

1. Gauze bandages, usually in rolls of 10 yards 1, 2, or 3 inches wide

2. Elastic bandages of woven material in various widths and lengths

3. Triangular bandages, usually of muslin, approximately 55 inches across at the base and from 36 to 40 inches along the sides (These bandages are included in first aid kits and are useful to cover large areas, as slings, and can be folded lengthwise as cravat bandages. They also can be folded into a thick pad for pressure over a wound to control hemorrhage. Triangular bandages are usually of muslin.)

4. A binder of muslin, to be applied to the chest or abdomen (A large towel or part of a sheet can substitute for a binder. A binder is rarely used except as an emergency bandage or dressing to cover a large area of the trunk, such as the chest or abdomen. It may be pinned in place or held with multiple ties or cravat bandages. Great care must be taken not to apply a binder so tightly that it interferes with breathing.)

5. Other emergency bandages (Can be devised from handkerchiefs, household linen, belts, ties, socks, or stockings. Bandages can be held in place with adhesive, plastic or masking tape, safety pins, or clips. Gauze and muslin bandages can be split and tied.)

III. COMBINATION DRESSINGS AND BANDAGES

Adhesive strips with an attached gauze dressing are available commercially in a wide variety of sizes and shapes. Another useful dressing-bandage combination is the bandage compress, which is usually included in the supplies of a first aid kit. It consists of a pad made of several thicknesses of sterile gauze sewed to the middle of a strip of gauze or muslin. Bandage compresses are the most useful and efficient combination of bandage and dressing to apply to a large wound as an emergency cover. The dressing portion provides bulk, over which pressure may be applied for control of severe hemorrhage.

IV. SPECIAL PADS

Large, thick-layered, bulky pads with an outer waterproofed surface are available in several sizes for rapid application to an extremity or to a large area of the trunk. Because they are often used in the treatment of victims with circular burns, they are sometimes called "burn pads" or "general purpose dressings."

V. APPLICATION OF BANDAGES

A. General principles

1. A bandage should be snug (it is useless if too loose), but not so tight as to interfere with circulation, either at the time of application or later if swelling occurs.

2. To ensure that circulation is not interfered with—

   a. Leave the person's fingertips exposed when a splint or bandage is applied to the arm, and leave the toes exposed when a splint or bandage is applied to the leg.

   b. Watch for swelling, changes of color, and coldness of the tips of fingers or toes, indicating interference with circulation.

   c. Loosen bandages immediately if the victim complains of numbness or a tingling sensation.

   d. Never apply a tight circular bandage about a person's neck; it may cause strangulation.

B. Elastic bandages

Although they are the easiest of all bandages to apply and are especially useful since they conform more readily to the injured part than gauze or muslin, they are the most hazardous because of the tendency of the first-aider to stretch them so much that circulation or nerve function may be impaired. They are rather expensive but can be laundered and used repeatedly for a number of purposes.

In using elastic bandages, the first-aider must take great care not to stretch the material too tightly.

C. Gauze bandages

1. Application

Skill is necessary in applying a gauze bandage to prevent

its slipping and stretching, because gauze is very loosely woven. Never apply a wet gauze bandage. It will shrink as it dries and become too tight. Gauze can be used to bandage almost any part of the body. Choose the appropriate width.

2. Most common uses

    a. Circular bandages

    b. Spiral bandages

    c. Figure-of-eight bandages (for joint areas)

    d. Fingertip bandages (formerly called recurrent)

D. Triangular bandages

Triangular bandages are useful as an emergency cover for the entire scalp, the hand or foot, or any large area. Such a bandage also is used as a sling for fracture or other injury of the arm or hand. Folded into a cravat bandage (*cravat* means necktie), the triangle can be used as a circular, spiral, or figure-of-eight bandage; it can be used, also, as a tie for a splint, as a constricting band, and as a tourniquet. If the cravat bandage is folded several times again to form a thick pad, it can serve as an emergency dressing for control of bleeding or can be placed over another dressing to provide protection and pressure.

E. Adhesive-strip dressings

Adhesive-strip dressings or homemade substitutes are used for small wounds following thorough cleansing. Blot the surface dry before applying the tape, and for a cut, hold the edges of the wound together as the dressing is secured in place.

F. Methods of applying bandages

1. Arm sling

Prepare a triangular piece of cloth approximately 55 inches across the base and from 36 to 40 inches along the sides. Regular triangular bandages of this size may also be purchased in unit packages.

    a. Place one end of the bandage over the uninjured shoulder and let the other end hang down in front of the chest, parallel to the side of the body.

b. Carry the point behind the elbow of the injured arm (Fig. 73A).

c. Carry the second end of the bandage up over the shoulder and tie the two ends together at the side of the neck—not over the spine (Figs. 73B and 73C).

d. Bring the point of the bandage forward and pin it to the front of the sling (Fig. 73D).

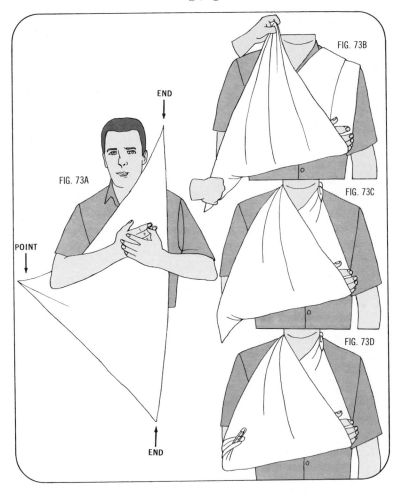

e. If a pin is not available, twist the point of the bandage until it is snug at the elbow and tie a single knot.

f. Make sure that the ends of the fingers extend just beyond the base, so that you can observe whether or not the circulation is cut off.

g. In all cases of injury to the hand or lower forearm, adjust the sling so that the hand is elevated 4 or 5 inches above the level of the elbow.

2. Triangular bandage folded as a cravat

To make a cravat, bring the point of a triangular bandage (Fig. 74A) to the middle of the base (74B). Then fold lengthwise along the middle until you obtain the desired width (Figs. 74C and 74D).

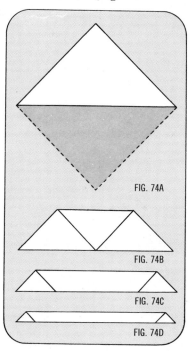

FIG. 74A

FIG. 74B

FIG. 74C

FIG. 74D

3. Triangular bandage for the scalp and forehead

Fold a hem about 2 inches wide along the base. Place compress. Put the dressing in place with the hem on the outside, place the bandage on the head so that the middle of the base lies on the forehead close down to the eyebrows and the point hangs down the back (Fig. 75A). Carry the two ends around the head above the ears and cross (do not tie) them just below the bump at the back of the head (Fig. 75B). Draw the ends snugly, carry them around the head, and tie them in the center of the forehead (Fig. 75C). Steady the head with one hand and with the other draw the point down firmly behind to hold the compress securely against the head. Pick up the point and tuck it in where the bandage ends cross (Fig. 75D) or pin it down with a safety pin at the back of the head.

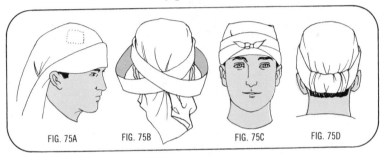

FIG. 75A   FIG. 75B   FIG. 75C   FIG. 75D

4. Cravat bandage for forehead, ears, or eyes

Place the center of the cravat over the compress that covers the wound (Fig. 76A). Carry the ends around to the opposite side of the head and cross them (Fig. 76B). Bring them back to the starting point and tie them (Fig. 76C).

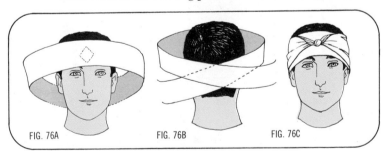

FIG. 76A   FIG. 76B   FIG. 76C

5. Cravat bandage for cheek or ear

Use a wide cravat. Start with the middle of the cravat over the compress that covers the cheek or ear (Fig. 77A). Carry one end over the top of the head and the other under the chin. Cross the ends at the opposite side, bringing the short end back around the forehead and the long end around the back of the head (Fig. 77B). Tie them over the compress (Fig. 77C). *Never* use the method for fracture of the jaw or where there is bleeding in the mouth or danger of vomiting, unless an attendant will be constantly present to loosen the bandage in an emergency.

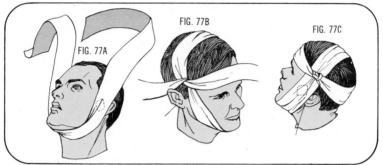

FIG. 77A

FIG. 77B

FIG. 77C

6. Cravat bandage for elbow or knee

Bend the elbow or knee at a right angle unless this movement produces pain. Use a rather wide bandage. Start with the middle of the bandage over the dressing at the elbow (Fig. 78A). Carry the ends around in opposite directions—one end around the upper arm or leg and the other end around the lower part—(Fig. 78B), crossing them in the hollow (Fig. 78C). Continue around, covering the dressing, back to the hollow and tie to the outside (Figs. 78D and 78E).

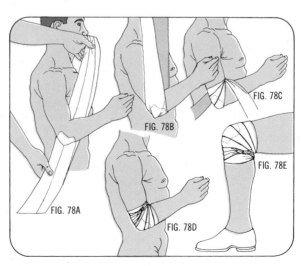

FIG. 78A

FIG. 78B

FIG. 78C

FIG. 78D

FIG. 78E

G. Anchoring a bandage

1. Place the end of the bandage on a bias at the starting point (Fig. 79).

2. Encircle the part, allowing the corner of the bandage end to protrude (Fig. 80).

3. Turn down the protruding tip of the bandage (Fig. 81) and encircle the part again (Fig. 82).

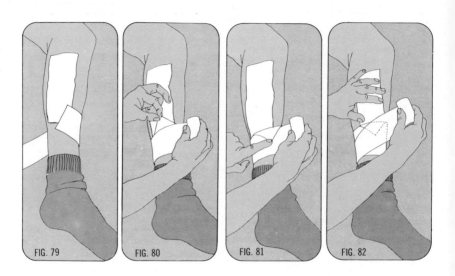

FIG. 79   FIG. 80   FIG. 81   FIG. 82

H. Tying off a bandage

Several ways to secure a bandage in place are listed on page 179, item 5. Another method to tie the gauze or muslin in place is as follows: Take the bandage end in a direction away from the body part being covered; loop around the thumb or finger and continue back to the opposite side of the body part (Fig. 83); encircle the part with the looped end and the free end and tie (Fig. 84).

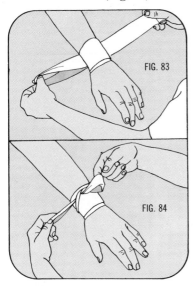

FIG. 83

FIG. 84

I. The circular turn

Circular turns simply encircle the part with each layer of bandage superimposed on the previous one. It is the simplest of all bandage turns. However, its use is limited to covering parts of uniform width, such as the toe and head.

J. Open and closed spiral bandage of the limb

Begin by anchoring as previously described (see Figs. 79 through 82, page 186); continue to encircle the area to be covered by the use of spiral turns spaced so that they do not overlap (Figs. 85 and 86); complete the bandage by tying off (Fig. 87). This bandage may be useful as a temporary ban-

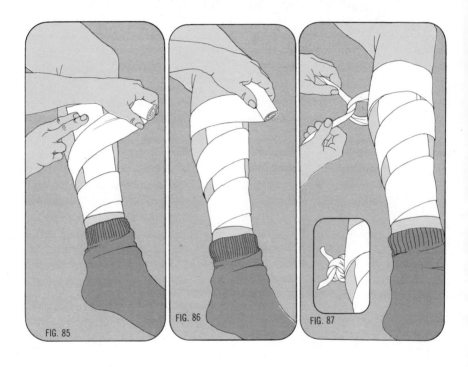

FIG. 85

FIG. 86

FIG. 87

dage, for splinting, and when used to hold a large burn
dressing in place. It may be closed (closed spiral) simply by
continuing to encircle with spiral turns until all gaps are
closed.

K. Figure-of-eight bandage for hand and wrist

Anchor the bandage with one or two turns around the palm
of the hand. Carry it diagonally across the front of the wrist
and around the wrist (Fig. 88A). Again carry it diagonally
across the front of the wrist, and back to the palm (Fig. 88B).
This figure-of-eight maneuver is repeated as many times as is
necessary to fix the dressing properly. Complete by tying off.

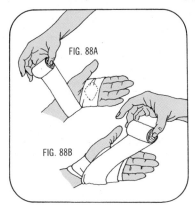

L. Fingertip bandage

This is a series of back and forth turns (Fig. 89A), called
recurrent turns, held in place by circular and spiral turns
(Figs. 89B and 89C). Secure by tying off (Fig. 89D). Normally
used to bandage fingers, the bandage may be adapted to
bandage the toes, scalp, or stumps of limbs. When areas such
as the scalp are to be covered, the next fold covers the
opposite side of the part being covered, and each succeeding
fold is worked toward the center until the area is sufficiently
covered. This bandage is held in place with circular turns.

Another method of securing this fingertip bandage is to use
the figure-of-eight turn to complete its application. From the
finger, or toe, take the end of the bandage diagonally across

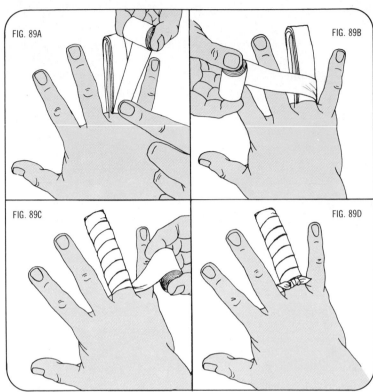

FIG. 89A

FIG. 89B

FIG. 89C

FIG. 89D

the back of the hand to the wrist; encircle one or more times (Fig. 90A); from the opposite side of the wrist, continue to the finger and loop (Fig. 90B). Repeat the figure-of-eight several times and tie off at the wrist (Fig. 90C).

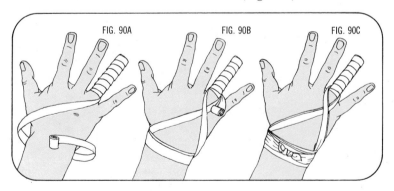

FIG. 90A   FIG. 90B   FIG. 90C

M. Figure-of-eight bandage for the ankle

Anchor the bandage on the instep and take two or three additional turns around the instep and foot. Carry the bandage diagonally upward across the front of the foot, then

around the ankle (Figs. 91A and 91B) and diagonally downward across the front of the foot and across under the arch.
Make several of these figure-of-eight turns, each turn overlapping the previous one by about two-thirds the width of the
bandage (Fig. 91C). Occasionally, use an extra turn around
the ankle. Complete by tying off (Fig. 91D).

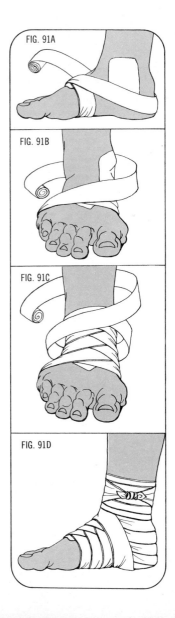

FIG. 91A

FIG. 91B

FIG. 91C

FIG. 91D

VI. FIRST AID KITS AND SUPPLIES

From your study of first aid you have learned how to improvise a number of bandages, dressings, and splints. It is, of course, more satisfactory to have sterile dressings, prepared splints, and other first aid equipment ready for use before an accident occurs.

There are two general types of first aid kits: (1) the unit type and (2) the cabinet type.

A. Unit-type kits

Unit-type kits have a complete assortment of first aid materials put up in standard packages of unit size or multiples of the unit size and arranged in cases containing 16, 24, or 32 units, with the 16- and 24-unit kits being the most popular. Each unit package contains one or more individual dressings. Each dressing is complete in itself and is sealed in a sterile wrapper. It contains just enough material to treat a single injury, thus eliminating waste. All liquids are put up in individual, sealed ampules, and consequently cannot deteriorate. There are no bottles to spill or break.

Illustrations and instructions for the use of the contents are on the front of each package. The desired unit packages are easy to locate, because the contents are clearly indicated on the top side in bold type. The unit packages fit like blocks in the case; they cannot shift or become disarranged. These types of kits are probably the most satisfactory for carrying in a car or truck or in a pack.

Standard refills are supplied by various manufacturers and can be changed easily to meet the needs of the purchaser. Unit refills are easy to obtain. The original cost may be slightly higher, but when materials are subject to much handling by many different persons, this type is generally cheaper and more satisfactory in the long run. There is no contamination or waste of unused materials. The kits can be obtained with contents selected to meet the particular needs of the purchaser.

1. Contents of 16-unit first aid kit

    2 units—1″ adhesive compress
    2 units—2″ bandage compress
    1 unit—3″ bandage compress

1 unit—4″ bandage compress
1 unit—3″ x 3″ plain gauze pads
1 unit—gauze roller bandage
2 units—plain absorbent gauze—1/2 sq. yd.
2 units—plain absorbent gauze—24″ x 72″
3 units—triangular bandages—40″
1 unit—tourniquet, scissors, tweezers

2. Contents of 24-unit first aid kit

2 units—1″ adhesive compress
2 units—2″ bandage compress
2 units—3″ bandage compress
2 units—4″ bandage compress
1 unit—3″ x 3″ plain gauze pads
2 units—gauze roller bandage
1 unit—eye dressing packet
4 units—plain absorbent gauze—1/2 sq. yd.
3 units—plain absorbent gauze—24″ x 72″
4 units—triangular bandages—40″
1 unit—tourniquet, scissors, tweezers

B. Cabinet-type Kits

Cabinet kits are made for a wide variety of uses and range in size from pocket versions to large industrial kits. They are made to accept packages in different shapes and sizes. Contents may be varied by the purchaser to suit his particular first aid needs. The extra space in most cabinet kits also allows additional items to be inserted according to user's needs.

Cabinet kits contain a large enough supply of most first aid items to be used for more than a single treatment. However, all sterile materials are individually wrapped.

Cabinet kits carry familiar first aid items that are easily recognized in an emergency. Although the different-size packages allow for some shifting of products in transported kits, they have the advantage of a functional package design that does not waste unnecessary space.

Refills are obtainable from most drugstores or through safety equipment distributors.

C. Other kits

Kits can be either purchased or can be assembled from improvised materials. All kits, whether purchased or improvised, are satisfactory if the following points are observed in their selections:

- The kit should be large enough and should have the proper contents for the place where it is to be used.
- The contents should be arranged so that the desired package can be found quickly without unpacking the entire contents.
- Material should be wrapped so that unused portions do not become dirty through handling.

Types and sizes of kits to meet specific needs should be selected and supplied with items recommended by your consulting physician.

14

BONE AND JOINT INJURIES

I. DEFINITIONS

Multiple injuries to the skeletal system, including the bones, joints, and ligaments, and to the adjacent soft tissues are common in all types of major accidents.

A. Fracture

A fracture is a break or crack in a bone.

1. Closed fractures

Closed (or simple) fractures are those not related to open wounds on the surface of the body (Fig. 92), although there may be a laceration over or near the fracture site.

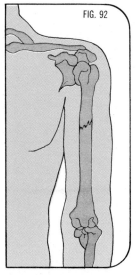

FIG. 92

2. Open fractures

Open (or compound) fractures are those associated directly with open wounds (Fig. 93). An open fracture may

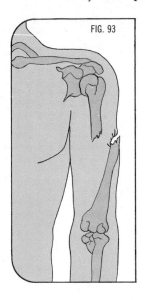

FIG. 93

result from external violence or may be produced by injury from within as broken ends of a bone protrude through the skin at the time of the accident or later through motion or mishandling of the fractured bone.

B. Dislocation

A dislocation is an injury to the capsule and ligaments of a joint that results in displacement of a bone end at a joint.

C. Fracture dislocation

A fracture dislocation is a dislocation associated with a fracture.

D. Sprain

A sprain is an injury to a joint ligament or a muscle tendon in the region of a joint. It involves the partial tearing or stretching of these structures, injuries to blood vessels, and contusions of the surrounding soft tissue without dislocation or fracture.

E. Strain

A strain is an injury to a muscle that results from overstretching. It may be associated with a sprain or a fracture.

II. FRACTURES

A. Causes

The most common causes of fractures are motor vehicle accidents, or accidents related to falls and recreational and sports activities. Some fractures result from very slight injuries, particularly in older people, because of brittle or abnormal bones.

B. Signs and symptoms

If an accident victim is conscious he will usually be able to provide clues to possible fractures. He may recall his position before the injury and relate what happened as he fell or struck some object. In addition—

- He may have heard or felt a bone snap.
- He may indicate the location of pain and tenderness and difficulty in moving the injured part.
- He may also report a grating sensation of broken bones rubbing together.
- He may report abnormal or false motion in an area of the body.

Other signs of fracture include—

- Differences in the shape and length of corresponding bones on the two sides of the body
- Obvious deformities
- Swelling
- Discoloration
- Pain or tenderness to touch

1. Closed fractures

Closed fractures are much more common than open fractures. As a rule, accurate diagnosis can be made only by a physician with the assistance of X-ray examination. The first aid worker should *suspect* that a bone is broken when any of the signs are present. Even if there is a doubt, to prevent aggravation of existing injuries, he should carry out first aid measures for a fracture.

2. Open fractures

In an *open* fracture, the wound usually is caused by a broken bone end that tears through the skin and, in most cases, slips back again. Sometimes the wound is caused by machinery or by a missile, such as a bullet that penetrates the skin and breaks the bone. Open fractures are much more serious because of tissue damage and bleeding and the danger of infection, because the fracture area is always contaminated.

C. Objectives

1. To provide all necessary first aid care

2. To keep the broken bone ends and the adjacent joints from moving

3. To give care for shock

D. First aid principles

1. To maintain an open airway and apply artificial respiration if indicated

2. To rescue, if necessary, and to protect against further injury

3. To call for an ambulance, if indicated, or medical assistance

4. To prevent motion of the injured parts and the adjacent joints

5. To elevate involved extremities, if possible, without disturbing the suspected fracture

6. To apply splints, if modern ambulance service is not available, if there is a delay in transportation, or in less serious injuries before seeking medical assistance for diagnosis and treatment

Do not attempt to set (or reduce) a fracture or try to push a protruding bone end back.

If splinting and transportation are necessary, the bone end may slip back when the limb is straightened for splinting.

If an ambulance or rescue squad can arrive within a short period after an accident, when an injured person obviously requires hospitalization, do not attempt to move the victim unless there is danger of fire, carbon monoxide poisoning, explosion, drowning, or other life-threatening emergencies. Above all, in attempting rescue, do not drag victims out of vehicles, or from under wreckage, or throw them on the ground in your haste to save their lives.

If possible, even in the midst of a crowded street or highway, take the time to tie a victim's injured leg to his uninjured one, or bind his injured arm to his chest or side.

Lift and move an unconscious victim as though there is injury to his neck or spine.

Wait for adequate help—at least three and preferably four persons—and obtain a rigid support for the victim's back, if possible.

Following a neck or spinal injury during water activity, float the victim to shore without bending his neck or back. *Do not* lift the victim out of the water without a back support.

Delegate others to telephone for an ambulance and the police, if necessary, and to assist in maintaining order in the area of the accident.

If an open fracture is evident or suspected, treat the wound as outlined previously:

1. Remove or cut away the victim's clothing.

2. Control hemorrhage by applying pressure through a large sterile (or clean) dressing over the wound.

3. Do not wash the wound, do not probe it, and do not insert your fingers into it.

4. If a fragment of bone is protruding, cover the entire wound with a large, sterile bandage compress or pads; if these are not available, use freshly laundered sheets or towels.

5. Do *not* replace bone fragments.

Apply splints, as described below, according to the location of the fracture. Then elevate the limb slightly to reduce hemorrhage and swelling. Open fractures should have priority over closed fractures for transportation and medical treatment, unless associated injuries dictate otherwise.

E. Splinting

Splints are devices applied to the arms, legs, or trunk to immobilize the injured part when a fracture is suspected. They decrease pain and the likelihood of shock by preventing motion of the broken bone ends and the adjacent joints. They also protect against further injury during transportation for medical treatment.

1. There are many types of splints available commercially. However, very satisfactory emergency splints can be made from corrugated cardboard (Fig. 94); newspapers, boards, straight sticks, rolled-up blankets, pillows, etc. A

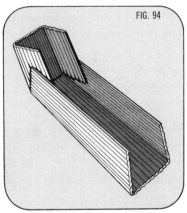

FIG. 94

simple splinting technique in an emergency is to tape or tie the injured leg to the uninjured one—with padding between, if possible—(Fig. 95); or to bind an injured

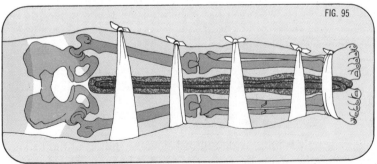

FIG. 95

arm, after padding, to the chest if the elbow is bent, or to the side if the elbow is straight.

2. The splint should be long enough to extend past the joints on either side of a suspected fracture.

3. The splint should be adequately padded between the splint and the skin, especially over bony places. The ends of board splints should also be well padded unless they extend beyond the body.

4. Splints may be held in place by strips of cloth torn from skirts or other material, large handkerchiefs, neckties, cravat bandages, or other similar material.

5. Joints should be immobilized above and below the location of the suspected fracture.

6. In fractures of the arm, check the pulse in the wrist and inspect the fingers frequently for swelling or bluish discoloration, which is a good indication that the bandages are too tight.

7. If the victim complains of numbness, tingling sensations, or inability to move his fingers or toes, loosen ties immediately—otherwise, permanent nerve damage may result. If splints are used in fractures of legs or feet and these symptoms appear, loosen the bandages, remove the victim's shoes and hose, and examine his toes repeatedly for color changes or swelling. If these signs appear, it may be necessary to further loosen bandages and reapply them.

8. It is important to remember that a person often can move parts below the break with little or no pain. It is also important to remember that he *should not move* the injured part.

9. Never test for fracture by having the victim move the part or try to walk on a possibly broken leg.

10. Do not allow an accident victim to move his head (or do not move it yourself) when there is a possible neck or spine injury. Movement may cause further damage to the spinal cord and result in paralysis.

11. If it is necessary to straighten and splint a deformed limb, proceed as follows:

    a. Place one hand above and one below the fracture to support it.

    b. Give care for shock.

    c. For fracture of the leg, have someone grasp the end of the limb and pull gently and steadily until splints are applied.

    d. Apply splints.

III. SPECIFIC FRACTURES

  A. Shoulder

    1. Fracture of the scapula

A fracture of the scapula (shoulder blade) is generally the direct result of the impact of a fall or an automobile collision. Dislocations of the shoulder joint, sprains, and contusions are common in this area. First aid consists of applying a sling and bandaging the victim's upper arm to his chest wall (Figs. 96A through 96F).

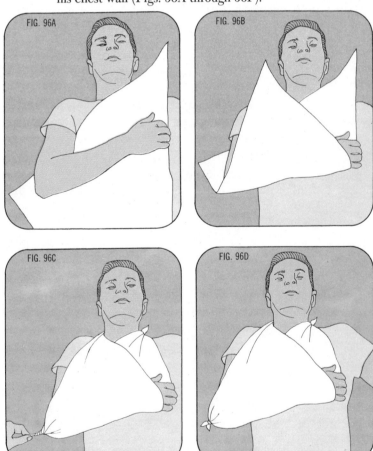

FIG. 96A   FIG. 96B

FIG. 96C   FIG. 96D

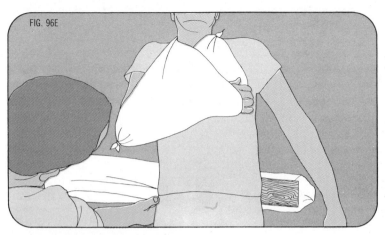

FIG. 96E

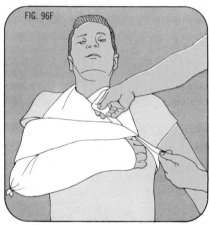

FIG. 96F

2. Fractures of the clavicle

Fractures of the clavicle (collarbone) usually occur in the weakest portion, which is one-third of the distance from the tip of the shoulder to the sternum. These fractures are particularly common with children and ordinarily heal without complication in 2 or 3 weeks (twice as long with adults). First aid consists of applying a sling to elevate the victim's arm and shoulder blade, which fall because of the loss of support from the clavicle, and then binding the arm to the victim's chest.

B. Humerus (the bone in the upper arm)

    1. <u>First aid</u> for a closed fracture

        Place a pad in the victim's armpit, apply a splint or improvised splint, tied in place above and below the break area (Fig. 97), and support his forearm with a sling that

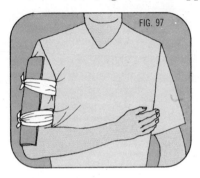

FIG. 97

        does not produce upward pressure at the fracture site (Fig. 98). Bind the victim's upper arm to his chest wall (Fig. 99).

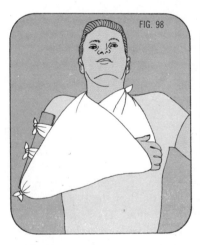

FIG. 98

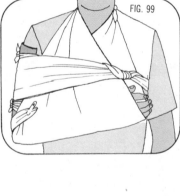

FIG. 99

    2. <u>First aid</u> for an open fracture

        Cover the wound with a large sterile, or clean, dressing and apply a splint that does not press against the area of the break. Do not attempt to cleanse the wound.

In the absence of a splint, support the victim's arm with a sling and bind it to his chest with an encircling bandage.

3. Immobilization

Remember that the *three places to immobilize* a fracture (or suspected fracture) of the upper arm are—

a. Broken bone ends

b. Shoulder

c. Elbow

C. Elbow

1. Location

Elbow fractures may involve the lower part of the humerus or the bones of the forearm.

2. First aid

a. Place the victim's forearm in a sling and bind it to his body. If the fracture occurred with the elbow straight, do not attempt to bend it to apply a sling. After placing a protective fold of cloth in the victim's armpit, secure a well-padded splint along both sides of the entire arm with ties.

b. Have the victim lie down and elevate his arm.

c. If a splint is not available, wrap a pillow about the arm, centering it at the elbow, and tie or pin the two sides together.

D. Forearm and wrist

1. Bones involved

The two bones of the forearm (ulna and radius) may be fractured individually or together.

2. First aid

Fractures in the midportion of the forearm and wrist are treated in the same way as fractures of the shaft of the humerus.

a. Immobilize the broken bone ends, the wrist and the elbow, by applying well-padded splints on each side (Figs. 100, 101A, and 101B).

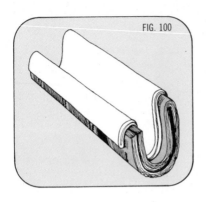

FIG. 100

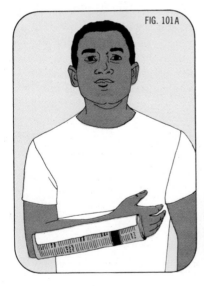

FIG. 101A

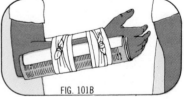

FIG. 101B

b. Bend the elbow and apply a sling with a slight elevation, keeping the thumb pointing upward (Fig. 102).

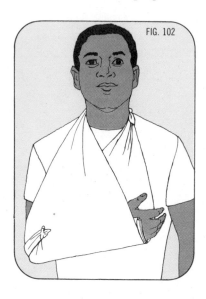

FIG. 102

E. Upper leg

1. Causes and characteristics

Fractures of the shaft of the femur usually result from falls or traffic injuries. The victim is in severe pain and shock, as a rule, and markedly disabled. The foot is characteristically turned outward and the limb shortened owing to overlapping of the bone ends due to muscular spasm.

2. First aid

a. If the victim is to be transported only a short distance on a stretcher, place a blanket between the legs and bind them together.

b. If you use improvised board splints, they should be well padded and should reach from the victim's armpit on the outer side and groin on the inner side to below his heel (Fig. 103).

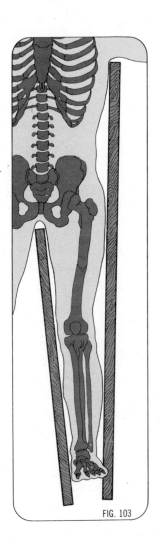

FIG. 103

c. To apply the board splint, assemble needed supplies (Fig. 104). Push the cravat bandages (or strips of cloth)

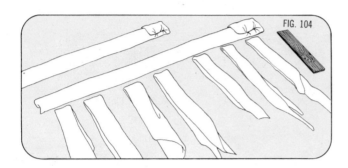

FIG. 104

under the victim at the body angles of the ankle, the knee, and the lower back. Slide bandages into place (Fig. 105). Place padded splints in position (Fig. 106).

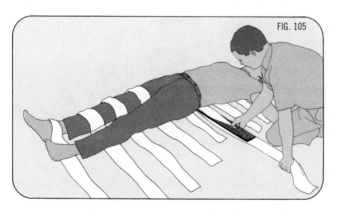

FIG. 105

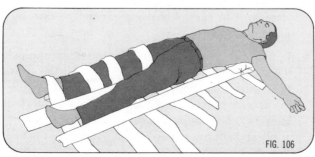

FIG. 106

Place additional padding at the knee and ankle. Complete by making snug ties on the outer splints (Figs. 107 and 108).

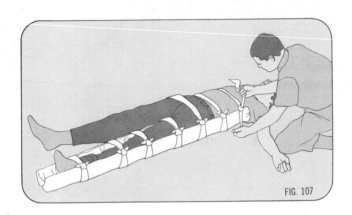

FIG. 107

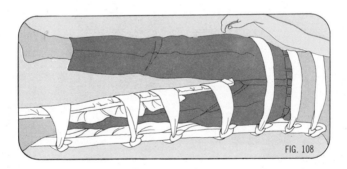

FIG. 108

d. If an open wound is present, do not attempt to cleanse it. Cover it with a sterile or clean bulky pad after cutting away contaminated clothing, apply pressure through it to control bleeding, secure the dressing in place, and splint.

e. If at all possible, a traction splint should be applied at the scene of the accident for fractures of the shaft of the femur. This splint will provide the best fixation of the fracture and will make the victim comfortable. However, *only* persons with specific training in the application of traction splints should attempt to apply the splint.

F. Kneecap

1. Causes and characteristics of fracture

The patella, or kneecap, is in front of the knee joint. It is fractured usually by a direct blow or in injuries sustained when control of the knee is lost, with the front thigh muscles pulling violently on the kneecap.

2. <u>First aid</u>

Apply a pillow splint about the knee or padded splints from below the victim's heel to his buttocks along the back of the leg, with the leg extended (Fig. 109).

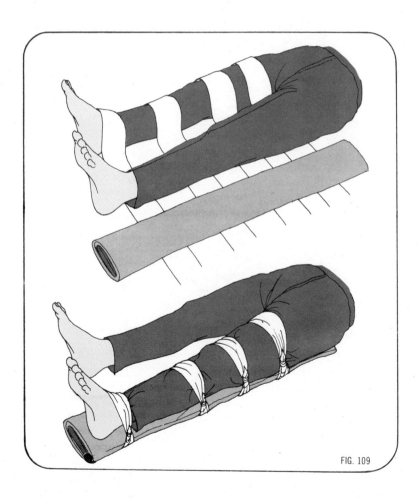

FIG. 109

G. Lower leg

1. Description

The bones of the lower leg are the tibia, or shinbone, which supports the weight of the body, and the fibula, which forms the outside wall of the ankle and is on the outer side of the leg.

2. First aid for fractures of the tibia and fibula

a. Apply well-padded splints on both sides of the leg and foot (Fig. 110).

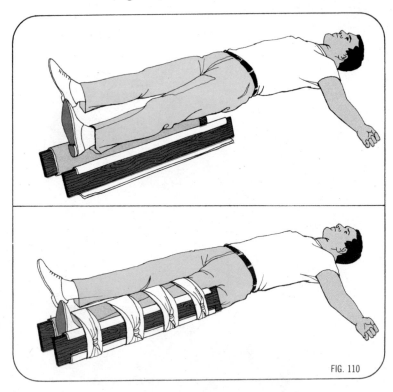

FIG. 110

b. In an emergency, insert blankets or towels between the legs and tie them together.

c. Remember to keep the victim's foot pointing upward, and check constantly to make sure that bandages do not interfere with the circulation to the lower leg and foot. Prevent movement of the broken bone ends, knee, and ankle.

H. Ankle and foot

   1. Description and causes

     The ankle is made up of the lower ends of the tibia and fibula, and the first bone of the foot (the talus). Fractures in this area occur most commonly in active sports, in falls, and in motor vehicle accidents.

   2. First aid

     a. Loosen or remove the victim's shoes (see page 201, item number 7) and hose and keep him lying down with his leg elevated.

     b. For an open wound, apply large, bulky dressings, sterile if possible.

     c. Splint with a pillow or blanket firmly applied, without attempting to correct the deformity (Fig. 111).

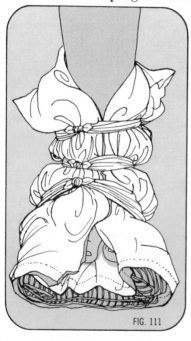

FIG. 111

I. Spine

   The backbone, or spinal column, is composed of 33 bones called vertebrae. The backbone encases the spinal cord, which passes through circular openings in the separate vertebrae. If a vertebrae or disk is fractured or dislocated, the spinal cord may be injured. Fractures of the neck or back are extremely dangerous, because the slightest movement may cause further damage to the spinal cord and result in paralysis.

1. <u>First aid</u> for fracture of the neck

    a. Do not allow the victim's head to be bent forward or backward, or to move from side to side. If the victim is having breathing difficulty, rescuers must follow the steps of airway control, the only modification being that head tilt should be minimal and forward displacement of the mandible and positive pressure breathing should be accomplished first if indicated.

    b. If the victim is lying on his back, a small pad or towel may be placed in the space under his neck. (Do not put a pillow under his head.)

    c. Place rolled-up clothing, blankets, or sandbags around the victim's head, the sides of his neck, and his shoulders to prevent movement.

    d. Anchor the restraining materials with bricks or stones, if available.

    e. Seek medical advice, and send for an ambulance with trained personnel.

2. <u>First aid</u> for fracture of the back

    a. Handle as little as possible.

    b. Send for an ambulance.

    c. Until help arrives, leave the victim in the position in which he was found, and unless there is delay in transportation or his condition is critical, take care of all other emergencies, such as breathing difficulty, hemorrhage, and open wounds, and apply dressings and splints as necessary.

    d. Do not twist the neck or back.

    e. Arrange rolled-up blankets or clothing on both sides of the trunk, head, and neck for immobilization.

    f. If a person with a fracture (or suspected fracture) of the back must be turned to obtain an open airway (for example, if he is face down in mud or water), make sure to obtain enough help so that the entire body is turned as a unit and no part twists or turns faster than other parts. Whenever possible, keep the victim in the position in which he was found.

IV. DISLOCATION

A dislocation is a displacement of a bone end from the joint, particularly at the shoulder (Fig. 112), elbow, fingers, or thumb

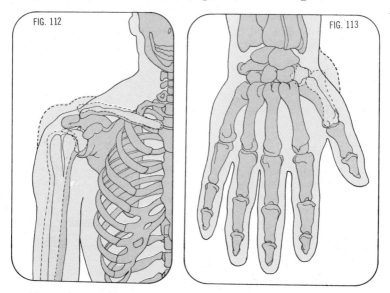

FIG. 112

FIG. 113

(Fig. 113), usually as a result of a fall or a direct blow. Unless given proper care, a dislocation may occur repeatedly.

    A. Signs of dislocation

      1. Swelling

      2. Obvious deformity

      3. Pain upon motion

      4. Tenderness to touch

      5. Discoloration

B. First aid

First aid should be essentially the same as for closed fractures:

1. Splint and immobilize the affected joint in the position in which it was found.

2. Apply a sling, if appropriate. Elevate the affected part, if a limb is involved.

3. Seek medical attention promptly.

4. *Never* attempt to reduce a dislocation, or to correct any deformity near a joint, since often extensive tearing of the joint capsule has occurred. Careless handling may cause additional tearing of supporting structures and, at the same time, may injure blood vessels and nerves in the area.

V. SPRAINS

A sprain is an injury to the soft tissue surrounding joints, usually as a result of forcing a limb beyond the normal range of a joint. The ligaments, muscles, tendons, and blood vessels are stretched or torn. The ankles, fingers, wrists, and knees are most often sprained.

A. Signs of sprain

1. Swelling

2. Tenderness

3. Pain upon motion

4. Discoloration

It is usually impossible to tell a sprain from a closed fracture without an X ray (for information on neck injuries, see page 214). Small chip fractures often accompany the tissue injuries of a sprain.

B. First aid

1. If the victim's ankle or knee is affected, do not allow him to walk.

2. Loosen or remove the victim's shoes (see page 201, item number 7), apply a pillow or blanket splint and elevate the victim's leg, because swelling may produce greater disability than the original injury itself (Figs. 114 through 116).

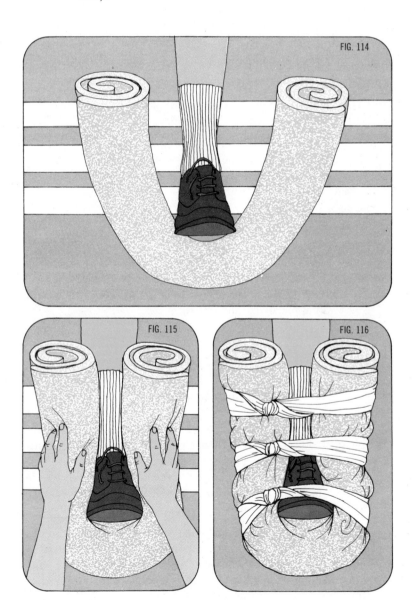

FIG. 114

FIG. 115

FIG. 116

3. In mild sprains, keep the injured part raised for at least 24 hours. (Do *not* soak in *hot* water.)

4. Apply cold, wet packs or place a small bag of crushed ice on the affected area, over a thin towel to protect the victim's skin. Packs may be applied over a period of several days. (Do *not* pack the joint in ice, and do *not* immerse the injured limb in water that contains ice.)

5. If swelling and pain persist, seek medical attention.

VI. STRAINS

A. Description and cause

Strains are injuries to muscles from overexertion. The fibers are stretched and sometimes partially torn. Back strains are commonly caused by improper lifting. (A person should lift with his legs and not his back.)

B. First aid

1. Bed rest, heat, and use of a board under the mattress for firm support is recommended for a person with a strained back.

2. Other strains are cared for by application of heat, warm, wet applications, and rest.

3. Medical care (All severe back strains should be seen by a physician.)

VII. PREVENTION OF ACCIDENTS RESULTING IN SKELETAL AND MUSCULAR INJURIES

When an impact force between any part of the body and some physical object is strong enough to overcome the structural strength of underlying bone, the bone either breaks or cracks. As in the case of wounds, impact forces that produce fractures involve motion of either man, a physical object, or both man and object.

Motor vehicle accidents and falling accidents are a major source of bone and joint or muscle tissue injury. Collision with fixed or other moving objects while engaged in such activities as running, skating, skiing, or cycling is also a common cause of fractures.

Prevention of skeletal and muscle tissue injuries requires that the source, direction, and amount of destructive impact forces be eliminated, controlled, or avoided. Many of the same conditions and activities that produce wounds, and the measures discussed in preventing wounds, are applicable to the bone, joint, and muscle accident problem.

The following discussion on prevention will limit itself to additional considerations regarding motor vehicle accidents, the more common conditions that may create falls, and those personal practices that help a person to avoid dislocations, sprains, and muscle strains.

A. Motor vehicle accidents

The death and bodily destruction caused each year in the United States by motor vehicle accidents presents what should be an intolerable situation for a civilized society. Almost half of all accidental deaths result from accidents that involve a motor vehicle.

Essentially, the problem is one of people, and its solution is the responsibility of people. A Red Cross course in first aid, with emphasis on accident prevention, will stimulate your thinking and should motivate you toward constructive action for greater highway safety and accident prevention. What follows is intended to provide a basis for discussion of the overall highway accident problem.

1. Driving skill and judgment

Driving skill and judgment cannot be separated; both are equally important in preventing accidents. Driving skill determines the ability of an individual to exercise physical control of a motor vehicle under normal as well as abnormal traffic, road, environmental, and other driving conditions. Driving judgment governs the ability of a driver to anticipate or recognize a potential accident condition or activity and to know what correction or evasive action can and must be taken to avoid an accident.

The effective exercise of both skill and judgment, however, is dependent upon the driver's attitude toward accident prevention. The motor vehicle driver who periodically ignores or simply refuses to accept responsibility for his own safety or the safety of others is, in reality, a licensed hazard to life and limb. Everything begins with attitude.

2. Vehicle condition

Like the human body, any machine is also subject to malfunction, occasionally needs remedial care, and should be given periodic checkups. A motor vehicle is a mass of moving parts, chambers, tubes, wires, electrical components, linkage, etc., that is subject to malfunction from friction, heat, chemical action, deterioration, and natural wear.

Since breakdown or malfunction of the vehicle can result in broken bones, bleeding wounds, or death, make certain that it is kept in good running condition. Follow the schedule of preventive maintenance suggested in your owner's manual. Learn to recognize sounds, odors, and vibrations that may be symptomatic of possible trouble. Check tires, windshield wipers, horn, and lights frequently; if defective, have them repaired or replaced immediately. Have a qualified automotive mechanic regularly inspect such items as brakes, wheel alignment, steering mechanism and linkage, and hydraulic, suspension, and exhaust systems.

3. Condition of the driver

Another contributing factor in motor vehicle accidents is the condition of the driver. As the nation's highways become more crowded, greater driving skill and judgment become necessary. Any condition that interferes with the normal skill and judgment of a driver increases the accident potential. Avoid any practice that may dull the senses, impair reaction time, or cloud mental alertness. Do not, for example, drive after drinking alcohol or after taking drugs that may cause you to become drowsy. Persons in a state of emotional tension or anxiety present a very dangerous accident hazard to themselves and others and should not be behind the wheel. Sources of distraction and irritability, such as a radio, overactive children, and the "backseat driver," should be kept under control. Fatigue is often a contributing factor in accidents. Take frequent rest stops on a long trip; and if fatigue impairs your alertness at any time, pull off the road and take a rest. Confirmed conditions also require corrective action; if you need glasses for driving, wear them.

4. Environmental conditions

Environmental conditions of snow, sleet, rain, fog, and darkness increase the danger of motor vehicle accidents occurring. Each of these conditions restricts visibility in varying degrees. Snow, sleet, and rain present the additional hazard of less than normal tire traction for controlling and stopping the vehicle.

Speed and distance between vehicles must be adjusted to prevailing conditions. On slippery streets or roads, avoid hard, sudden braking. Use a lower transmission gear so that the motor can help to slow the vehicle down, and if the brake must be used, pump it gently. Snow tires, chains, tire studs, and other gripping devices enhance control of a vehicle on snow- or ice-covered roads. Remember also to keep the windshield clean, and other windows as clear of ice and snow as possible.

5. Pedestrian safety

About two-thirds of all pedestrian accident fatalities and injuries occur to people crossing over or entering upon streets. Drivers, therefore, should exercise special caution near schools, churches, playgrounds, parking lots, pedestrian crosswalks, and on narrow residential streets where someone may walk into the path of a moving vehicle from behind a parked car.
Pedestrians can protect themselves by crossing streets only at intersections or marked crosswalks and by obeying traffic signals. If there is no sidewalk, stay on the left and walk facing traffic. At night, wear or carry something white; strips of reflecting tape on a raincoat help a driver to see you when inclement weather obstructs normal visibility.

B. Falling accidents

Falls are the second leading cause of accidental death,

ranking behind motor vehicle fatalities and ahead of fire and burn fatalities. About three out of every four deaths from falls happen to people 65 years of age or older. The majority of accidental falls occur in the home environment.

C. Slipping and tripping hazards

Wipe up spilled liquids on kitchen, bathroom, or other bare floor surfaces as soon as noticed. Use a nonslip floor wax. Make certain that small rugs are secured in some way and keep them away from the top and bottom of a stairway. Clean snow off steps and sidewalks, and use salt or sand on icy walk areas. Place a safety mat in the bathroom tub, or better yet, install handholds. Be careful of any play or work in wet grass, particularly if the work involves pushing a power mower.

Torn sections and rolled-up edges of carpets present a common tripping hazard. Brooms, vacuum cleaner hoses, small footstools, toys, tools, and similar objects left haphazardly on floors or stairs are all obstacles. Stairs should be well lighted, carpets or stair treads kept in good repair, and handrails installed for their entire length. Carelessly mislaid toys, garden tools, and other objects hidden in grass, or holes dug by children and animals present tripping hazards out of doors. Pegs and wires holding up young trees and shrubs create a hazard as well.

D. Climbing and reaching

Makeshift devices such as chairs or boxes provide an unsafe substitute for a sturdy stepladder. Reposition a ladder instead of taking the chance of overreaching. As a rule, keep your hips between the ladder rails. Use both hands when climbing a ladder, and face the ladder when climbing up or down. Make necessary arrangements for hoisting tools or paint before leaving the ground.

Ladder rails and rungs should be inspected before use. Because paint hides structural defects, do not paint ladders. A straight ladder should be firmly based, with its foot a quarter of the ladder length away from the wall. It is usually best to have a qualified expert do work involving considerable height, such as installing a television antenna. If you must perform any roof operations, use a safety belt and strong rope.

E. Special precautions

Remember, falls are the leading cause of accidental death and injury to older people. Older persons should avoid sudden head or body movements that may cause them to lose balance and should slow down when moving about from place to place. Stairs are particularly dangerous, since the balance, agility, and visual acuity and perception of older people are not as great as in youth.

One of the more frequent causes of physical injury to infants is falling from tables and bassinets. Make certain that infants are not left unattended in places where they might fall, even for a moment.

F. Joint and muscle tissue injury prevention

Dislocations result from too much stress on a joint. Injury-producing conditions are similar to those causing fractures, and the same type of prevention considerations can serve to eliminate, control, or avoid dislocations.

Sprains overstretch or tear either the ligaments of a joint or muscle tendons from their attachment to the skeleton. Weight thrown forcibly upon a joint, or sudden force that causes the joint to turn or twist from its normal range of movement, are common causes. While proper strapping or taping prior to participation in athletic activities help control the incidence of such injuries, the frequency of ankle and knee joint injuries in some sports serves to point up man's limited capabilities for preventing tissue and capsule injury to these joints. Head restraints in automobiles offer some measure of protection against neck sprains, commonly called "whiplash" injuries, which result from rear-end vehicle collisions.

Muscle strains most frequently involve the back muscles, and are usually the result of lifting too much weight, or lifting a heavy weight improperly. To avoid back strain when a heavy object must be lifted, observe the following precautions:

- Plant the feet firmly and apart.

- Squat—do not lean—forward, keeping the back as straight as possible, and get a good grip on the object.

- Lift slowly, pushing up with the strong thigh and leg muscles.

- Do not jerk the object upward or twist the trunk of your body as lifting takes place.

- To lower a heavy object, reverse the above procedure.

15

EMERGENCY RESCUE AND
SHORT-DISTANCE TRANSFER

Emergency rescue and transfer deal with the movement of victims away from hazardous locations and the use of protective methods to support a victim's body during emergency transfer.

Involvement of the first-aider in emergency rescue and transfer is limited to situations in which professional ambulance or rescue personnel and equipment are not or will not be available, to assisting those professionals when they are available, and to removing victims when there is immediate danger to their lives.

If a person is ill or injured to the extent that he will require transport to a medical facility, the first decision to be made by the first-aider is whether it is necessary for the victim to be transferred a short distance before being placed on a litter and in an ambulance. Unless there is immediate danger to the life of the victim from such hazards as those listed below, he should not be transferred until such life-threatening problems as airway obstruction and hemorrhage are cared for, wounds are dressed, and fractures are splinted.

It should be recognized that more harm can be done through improper rescue and transportation than through any other measures associated with emergency assistance. In the majority of situations, rescue from confinement or pinning should be carried out by ambulance or rescue personnel. Pending their arrival, the first-aider should gain access to the victim, give him emergency care, reassure him, and avoid ill-advised or foolhardy attempts at rescue that might jeopardize the safety of the victim as well as that of the first-aider.

I. DEFINITION OF EMERGENCY RESCUE

Emergency rescue is a procedure for moving a victim from a dangerous location to a place of safety.

II. INDICATIONS FOR IMMEDIATE RESCUE

A. Fire, danger of fire, or explosion
B. Danger of asphyxia due to lack of oxygen or due to gas
C. Serious traffic hazards
D. Risk of drowning
E. Exposure to cold or intense heat or to intense weather conditions
F. Possibility of injury from collapsing walls or building
G. Electrical injury or potential injury
H. Pinning by machinery

III. PROCEDURE

A. When it is necessary to remove victims from a life-threatening situation, the first-aider must—

1. Avoid subjecting the victim to any unnecessary disturbances

2. Ensure an open airway and administer artificial respiration if it is needed

3. Control bleeding

4. Check for injuries

5. Immobilize injured parts prior to movement of the victim, if possible

6. Arrange for transportation

B. It is difficult for inexperienced helpers to lift and carry a person gently. They need careful guidance. If there is time, it is wise to rehearse the lifting procedure first, using a practice subject. Other factors to be considered:

1. If you must lift someone to safety before a check for injuries can be made, protect all parts of the body from the tensions of lifting.

2. Support the arms and legs, the head, and the back. Keep the entire body in a straight line and keep it from moving.

3. Sometimes, although a checkup can be made, an injured part cannot be immobilized until the victim has been moved a short distance. If a limb is injured, place one

hand just above the injured area and one just below it. While helpers lift the body and another helper keeps the adjacent joints from moving, keep the injury from bending and twisting.

4. Any transfer is harmful unless the injured parts are immobilized. "Splint them where they lie," unless there is urgent danger.

5. It is usually best to wait until an ambulance is available. People who may have head injuries, fractures of the thigh, leg, and pelvis, or back injuries *should not be transported sitting up.* The injured parts need immobilization and the victim should be transported lying down, with the first-aider giving particular attention to maintaining an open airway at all times.

IV. METHODS OF TRANSFER

A. Immediate rescue without assistance

1. Pulling the victim

If a person must be pulled or dragged to safety, he should be pulled in the direction of the long axis of his body, preferably from the shoulders, not sideways (Fig. 117). Every effort must be made to *avoid bending* or twisting

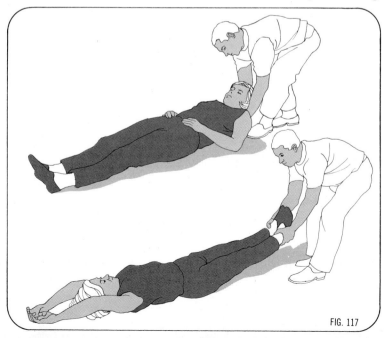

FIG. 117

his neck or trunk. The danger is less if a blanket or similar object (such as a small rug or a piece of cardboard) or a board, can be placed beneath him so that he can "ride" the object (Fig. 118). Do not try to lift or carry an injured

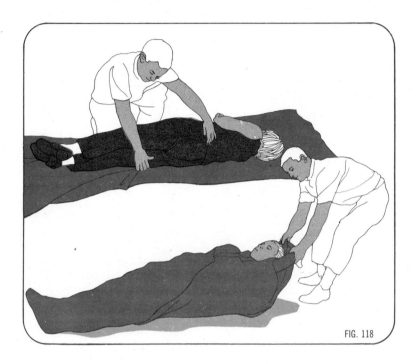

FIG. 118

person before a check for injuries can be made, unless you are sure that there is no major fracture or involvement of his neck or spine.

2. Lifting the victim

A lightweight adult or a child who has no serious wounds or skeletal injuries may be carried by one person. Place one hand under his knees and the other under his upper back and armpit for support (Fig. 119).

3. Supporting the victim

A person who has no serious wounds or skeletal injuries, who has not had a heart attack, and who is conscious may be assisted to walk to safety. Help him to his feet, place one of his arms around your neck, hold his hand at your

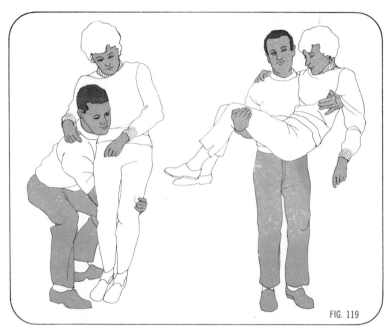

FIG. 119

chest (or shoulder) level, and place your other arm about his waist for additional support (Fig. 120). An assistant may be used, if available (Fig. 121).

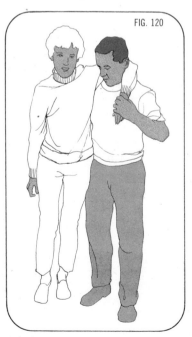

FIG. 120

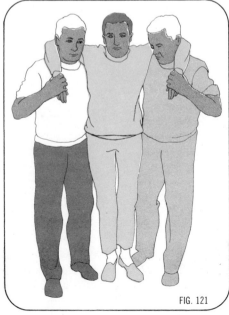

FIG. 121

B. Immediate rescue with assistance

Sometimes, the hazards are so great that it is necessary to move an injured person a short distance without first immobilizing the affected parts. If the victim is to be lifted by several persons, the first aid worker should devote himself to the area of greatest injury, protecting it as much as possible. He should prevent bending and twisting of injured parts, such as the limbs, by placing one of his hands just above and on top of the suspected injury and the other just below and under the part, as helpers lift the victim and support the main weight of the limb.

1. Chair carry

If a second person is available to assist, but no litter or blanket is available, a convenient technique for carrying a person is to seat him on a strong chair (Figs. 122 and 123). This method is also satisfactory for going up and down stairs, through narrow corridors, and around corners. This technique is not suitable for persons with neck or back injuries or injuries of the legs.

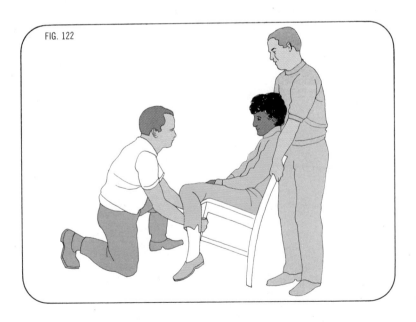

FIG. 122

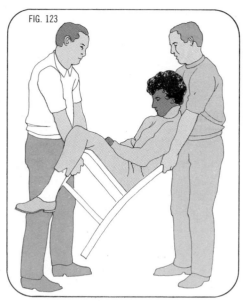

FIG. 123

2. Fore-and-aft carry

The fore-and-aft carry is a two-man technique. It may be used in moving an unconscious person but it is not applicable when there are serious injuries of the trunk or there are fractures (Figs. 124 and 125).

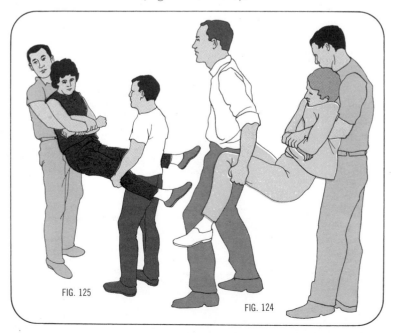

FIG. 125

FIG. 124

3. Two-handed and four-handed seats

Another two-man rescue technique is the two-handed seat or swing (Figs. 126 through 129). If the victim has no

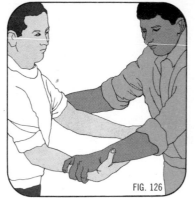

FIG. 126

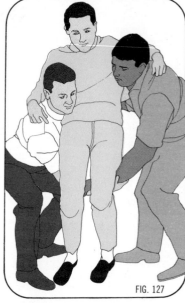

FIG. 127

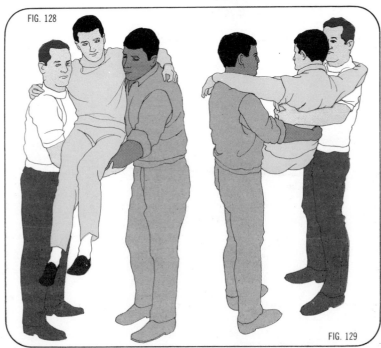

FIG. 128

FIG. 129

serious injuries and is able to cooperate with his rescuers, he may be placed on a two-handed seat, as shown, with his arms about the necks of the first aid workers and his back supported by their free hands, or the four-handed seat may be used (Fig. 130), in which case better support

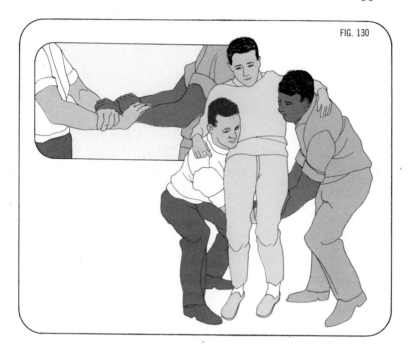

FIG. 130

is provided for seating, but the victim's back is not supported.

C. Blanket techniques

If transfer is necessary before a litter can be provided, a blanket can be placed under a person for lifting and carrying him a short distance. A blanket should never be used if there is a suspected fracture of the neck or back, unless the hazard is so great that time does not permit procuring a backboard. If the use of a blanket is necessary, one first aid worker should steady the victim's head, holding traction in a straight line away from his trunk. If his body is to be turned, it is moved as a unit so that no twisting or side-to-side motion of his neck or back occurs.

1. Placing blanket under victim from the side

Allow about two-thirds of the blanket to fall in folds or pleats beside the victim. Then place the folded (not rolled) portion snugly against his body (Fig. 131). Grasp the victim at his hips and shoulders and roll him gently about one-eighth of a turn away from the blanket (Fig. 132). Push the folded part of the blanket as far under the victim as possible and roll him back over the folds and approximately one-eighth of a turn in the opposite direction. Pull the blanket on through (Fig. 133). This procedure places

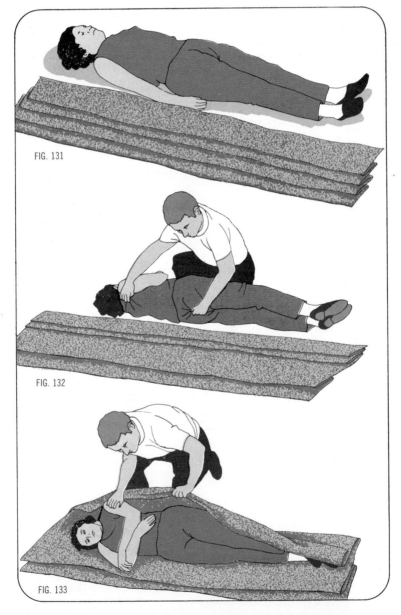

FIG. 131

FIG. 132

FIG. 133

the victim in the middle of the blanket, which can then be rolled from the sides and used to lift him onto a stretcher or to carry him to safety (see below). If others are available to assist, they should be used. (Figs. 134 and 135).

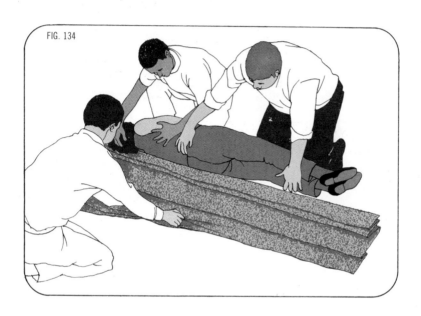

FIG. 134

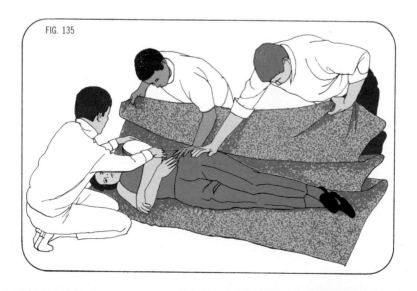

FIG. 135

2. Blanket lift

    a. Roll the blanket tightly at the sides until it fits the contours of the victim's body (Fig. 136).

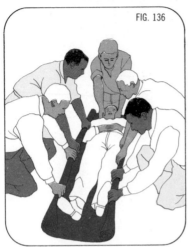

FIG. 136

    b. Two persons at the victim's shoulders grasp the blanket with their top hands at his shoulders and their bottom hands at his lower back. The two persons at the lower part of his body grasp the blanket with their top hands at his hips and their lower hands at the legs, just below the knees. No. 1 is at the victim's head, holding slight traction (Fig. 137).

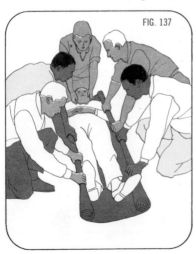

FIG. 137

c. At a signal, the persons holding the blanket lean back (away from the victim), using their back muscles and body weight. This action lifts the victim from 6 to 8 inches from the floor or ground so that a litter can be slid underneath (Fig. 138). The same procedure is used when a victim is in a prone position.

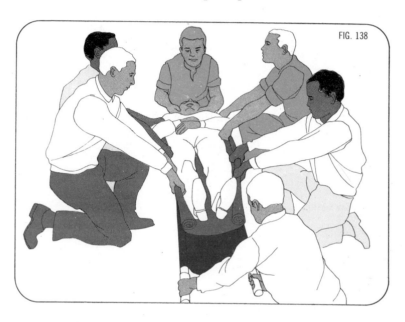

FIG. 138

d. All parts of the victim's body should be supported—the extremities, the head, and the trunk—and the victim's entire body should be kept immobile and in a straight line. Helpers should lift gradually, following the proper lifting instructions as given, so that they themselves will not suffer back injury. They also should guard against losing their balance. In all lifts, the leader should give appropriate preparatory signals prior to the actual signal for action so that all move as a unit; for example: "Prepare to lift!" and then "Lift!" or "Prepare to stand!" and then "Stand!"

D. Three-man hammock carry

This technique may be used with the victim on his back (supine) or on his face (prone). In either case, keep his chin up to maintain an open airway.

1. Victim in supine position

   a. Each carrier kneels on his knee that is closer to the victim's feet.

   b. No. 1 cradles the victim's head and shoulders with his top arm. His other arm is placed under the victim's lower back.

   c. No. 2, on the opposite side from No. 1, slides his top arm under the victim's back *above* No. 1's bottom arm and his other arm just below the victim's buttocks.

   d. No. 3 slides his top arm under the victim's thighs, above No. 2's bottom arm. His other arm is placed under the victim's legs below the knees (Fig. 139).

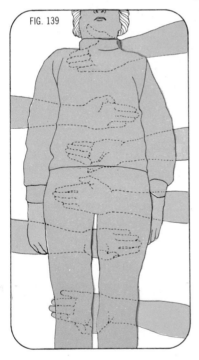

FIG. 139

NOTE. The hands of carriers No. 1 and No. 2 should be placed about halfway under the victim's body at this stage.

   e. The command "Prepare to lift!" is followed by the command "Lift!" and the victim is lifted to the carriers' knees and rested there while their hands are slid far enough under the victim to allow rotation of their hands *inward* to secure two interlocking grips (Figs. 140 and 141).

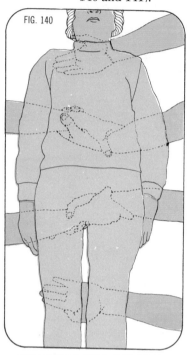

FIG. 140

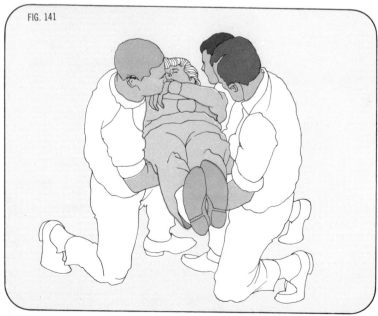

FIG. 141

f. The command "Prepare to stand!" is followed by the command "Stand!" and all carriers stand erect with the victim (Fig. 142).

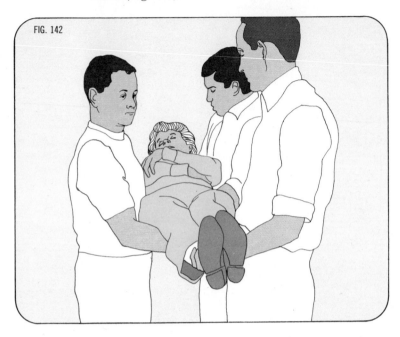

FIG. 142

To lower the victim to the ground or onto a litter, reverse the procedure.

2. Victim in prone position

The principles explained above should be used when the victim is in a prone position.

E. Three-man or four-man lift

1. Three bearers take up positions on one side of the victim and facing him, one at his shoulder, one at his hip, and one at his knees. If one side is injured, the three bearers should be on the uninjured side. A fourth bearer, if available, takes a position on the opposite side, at the victim's hip.

2. Each bearer kneels on his knee that is closer to the victim's feet. Then, simultaneously, the bearer at the victim's

shoulder puts one arm under the victim's head, neck, and shoulder, and the other under the upper part of the victim's back. Each bearer at the victim's hips places one arm under the victim's back and the other under his thighs. The bearer at the victim's knees places one arm under the victim's knees and the other under his ankles (Fig. 143).

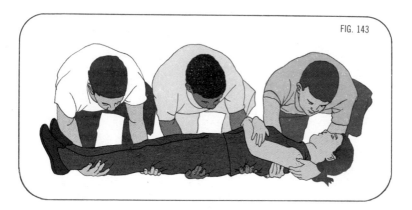

FIG. 143

3. The command "Prepare to lift!" is followed by the command "Lift!" and immediately all the bearers lift together and place the victim in line on their knees (Fig. 144).

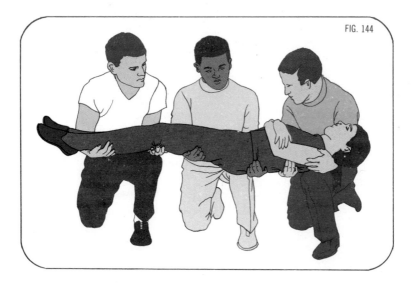

FIG. 144

4. If there is a fourth bearer, he places a stretcher under the victim and against the toes of the three kneeling bearers. The command "Prepare to lower!" is followed by the command "Lower!" and the victim is gently lowered to the stretcher.

To unload a stretcher, the rescuers reverse the procedure. The method described above is also used to place a victim in bed.

When it is necessary to transport a victim in a confined area, he may be carried by three bearers. The victim would then be rolled toward them (Fig. 145).

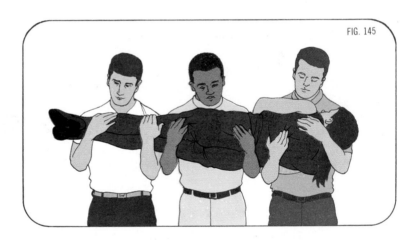

FIG. 145

F. Six-man lift and carry

There are three bearers on each side of the victim. Each kneels on his knee that is closer to the victim's feet. The bearers' hands, wrists, and forearms are worked gently under the victim until the palms of their hands are about at the midline of the victim's back (or stomach). The hands should be alternated from the two sides. The two hands under the victim's head may have the fingers interlocked to form a cup for his head (Figs. 146 and 147).

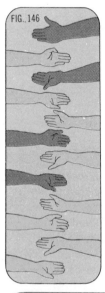

FIG. 146

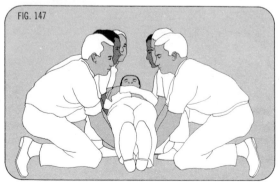

FIG. 147

The command "Prepare to lift!" is followed by the command "Lift!" and the victim is lifted on the bearers' hands and forearms to their knees. They must be careful to keep the victim's body in a straight line (Fig. 148). The command

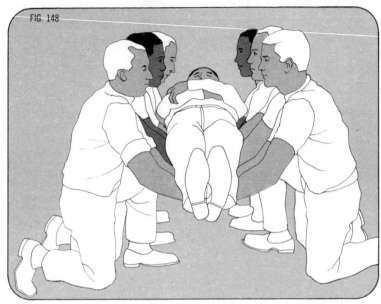

FIG. 148

"Prepare to stand!" is followed by the command "Stand!" and all bearers stand erect (Fig. 149). To lower the victim to the ground or onto a litter, reverse the procedure. If needed, additional bearers can be placed on both sides of the victim to assist in lifting.

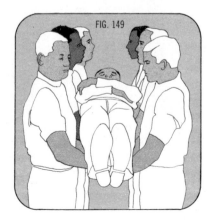

FIG. 149

G. Stretchers and litters

Of the litters shown, the "army litter" is most satisfactory for general use (Figs. 150A through 150D). In opening it, lock the bracing bars with your foot, if you are wearing shoes (Figs. 150B and 150C) or with the palm of your hand, not by grasping the bar with your hands and fingers. Before using the litter for the victim, test it by lifting someone at least as heavy as the victim.

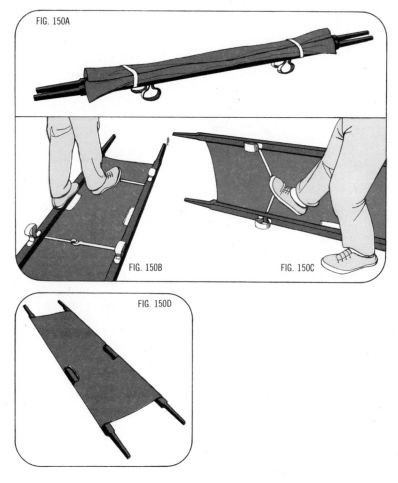

FIG. 150A

FIG. 150B

FIG. 150C

FIG. 150D

1. Improvised litter

In an emergency in which ambulance service is delayed or is not available, or in remote areas where litters or back-

boards are not available, an improvised litter may have to
be used to transport a person either to shelter or to a
source of transportation to a medical facility. A litter may
be improvised from clothing, a rug, or a blanket placed
over poles (Fig. 151). If available, a lightweight canvas

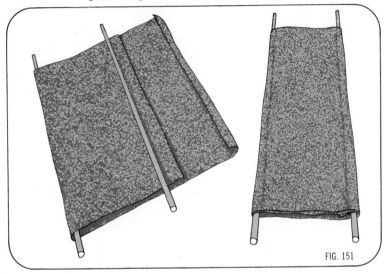

FIG. 151

lounge chair, an ironing board, a leaf from a table, or a
door may be used. An automobile seat is long enough for a
child. Near water, such things as floats, surfboards, and
water skis, as well as planks, may be used. Wheeled vehicles can sometimes be used to assist with an emergency
litter, and other means of transportation may be utilized.
If an ambulance or rescue vehicle can be brought to the
scene, and hazards do not demand transfer, it is better to
wait for the proper equipment.

2. Carrying techniques

   Care must be taken to secure the injured person or invalid
   properly, so that he will not roll or slide during transportation. If a neck fracture is suspected, additional padding is
   necessary to support the victim's head and neck. Use
   cravat bandages or other improvised ties.

3. Positions of bearers

   It is preferable to have four bearers: one at the victim's

head, one at his feet, and one at each side, all facing the direction of intended movement (Fig. 152). Each side bearer holds the side of the litter with his hand that is closer to the victim. All assume the proper lifting stance, and at the command "Lift!" all stand erect.

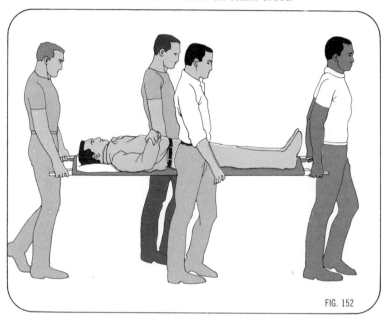

FIG. 152

At the command "March!" the bearer at the head of the litter steps off on his right foot, and the bearers at the sides and feet step off on their left feet. To lower the litter, the bearers reverse the steps used to lift the litter.

H. The vehicle transfer

The first-aider must protect victims of accidental injury or serious illness who require vehicle transfer on a litter against hasty or ill-advised transfer in trucks, station wagons, or any vehicles other than ambulances. On rare occasions, a toboggan or a substitute motor vehicle may be the only means of transport to a site accessible to ambulances. The drive should be at moderate speeds, with gentle stops and starts and with observation of all safety rules. However well-splinted or otherwise immobilized an injured part may be, a fractured or otherwise injured area sustains some harmful effect from the constant swaying and jolting of the vehicle as it rounds turns, slows down, increases speed, or encounters dips and elevations.

Accident victims often benefit from a period of rest before transfer. If the subject is ill, rather than injured, the first-aider customarily has no special preparation responsibilities unless delegated by a physician. Too often, a victim is subject to disturbing and exhausting preparation before transportation is begun.

It is most important to remember that people who may have head injuries, fractures of the thigh, leg, arm, or pelvis, or possible back injuries and those with heart attacks or chest or abdominal injuries should not be transported sitting up in automobiles. The injured parts need immobilization; the victim should be recumbent on a comfortable support; and he should be transported safely.

I. Rescues involving electrical emergencies with home appliances

Electrocution is common in the home from low voltage current. The danger in the home is often underestimated, especially the danger to the rescuer if he touches the same equipment or the injured person. The rescuer should disconnect the attachment plug from its socket or throw the main house electrical switch if possible. It may be necessary to separate the victim from the contact by utilizing a long, very dry pole, a dry rope, or length of dry cloth. Be sure that your hands are dry and that you are standing on a dry surface.

J. Toxic or oxygen-deficient atmospheres

First-aiders should not attempt rescues from toxic or oxygen-deficient atmospheres unless the area has been thoroughly ventilated or they have proper equipment for respiratory protection.

A room filled with gas can explode if someone turns on a light, rings the doorbell or telephone, or lights a match.

If you attempt to save someone in a gas-filled room, first shut off all the gas and electricity for the building. If there is no fire or smoke, open the windows and doors. This action will allow the gas to blow away.

Carbon monoxide poisoning is another example of toxic atmosphere that is extremely dangerous. If you rescue someone who has been poisoned by exhaust gases, remember that the poisonous gas can knock you out suddenly. Always ventilate the area before doing anything else, then remove the victim to fresh air and give all necessary first aid.

K. Rescues involving fires

If you are trapped in a burning building (or must enter to rescue someone), put a thick, wet cloth over your mouth and nose. This cloth will protect your air passages from the heat. It will not, however, protect you from the poisonous gases.

Before opening a door in a burning building, feel the door to check for extreme heat. If the door is very hot, try to find another way out.

If the door is cool (or slightly warm), crouch low behind the door as you open it slowly.

Usually the stairway is safer than the elevator when you are escaping from a burning building. The fire may damage the elevator and trap you inside.

If you are trapped on an upper floor, find a room with a window in it. Close the door and transom; open the window *slightly* and breathe the incoming air; signal for help by hanging something large (coat, sheet, rug) out of the window; then lie on the floor.

L. Water rescue

1. General information

Most drownings occur within reach of safety; rescue is, hence, often possible even if the first-aider is unable to swim.

2. Procedure

A swimming rescue should *not* be attempted except by someone trained in lifesaving. Additional information can be found in the American Red Cross textbook *Lifesaving and Water Safety,* which also includes a section on ice-accident prevention and rescue.

a. If a swimmer is in trouble near the dock or the side of a pool, lie down and extend your hand or foot to him; or

hold out a towel, shirt, stick, fishing pole, float, deck
chair, tree branch, or other object at hand and pull him
to safety (Figs. 153A through 153C). Use a line or ring

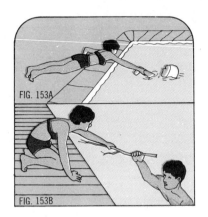

FIG. 153A

FIG. 153B

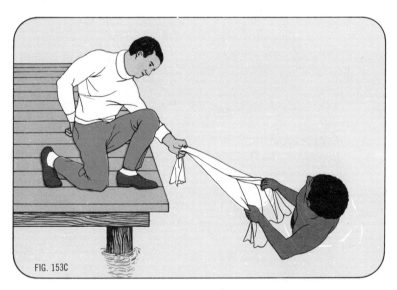

FIG. 153C

buoy, if possible (Fig. 154). If the swimmer is too far
from shore for these measures, wade into waist-deep
water first with a suitable object to extend to him, or

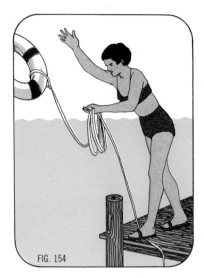

FIG. 154

push out a board to which he can cling while you go for help (Fig. 155A), or grasp his wrist and pull him to safety (Fig. 155B).

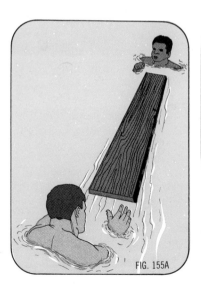

FIG. 155A

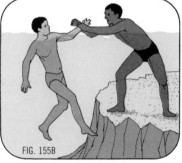

FIG. 155B

b. If a rowboat is available, row out to the victim and let him grasp the stern, or extend an oar and draw him around to the stern where he can hang on while you row to shore. If he is unable to hold onto the stern or the oar, pull him to the boat (Fig. 156), and, after checking for injuries, pull him into the boat.

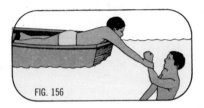

FIG. 156

c. Persons who drown usually die from lack of air and not from water in the lungs or stomach. Do not try to get water out of a victim. Start artificial respiration right away, whether you are in a boat, supporting the victim at the side of a boat, pulling him ashore, or on the shore.

d. As soon as the victim is able to breathe for himself, give him care for shock and get medical assistance.

M. Ice rescue

1. A useful device for ice rescue is a light ladder, from 14 to 18 feet long, with a light, strong line attached to the lowest rung.

2. The ladder should be shoved out on the ice to the limit of its length, and the cord will serve as an extension.

3. The rescuer may crawl out on the ladder to assist the victim (Fig. 157) if necessary. If the ice breaks under the ladder, the ladder will angle upward from the broken ice area and can be drawn to safety by other persons.

4. Other usable rescue devices are buoys, ropes, sticks, poles, and even a human chain of rescuers lying prone on the ice.

5. Victims of skating accidents who fall through the ice may

require artificial respiration, which should be administered on the way to shelter, as well as warming and treatment for shock.

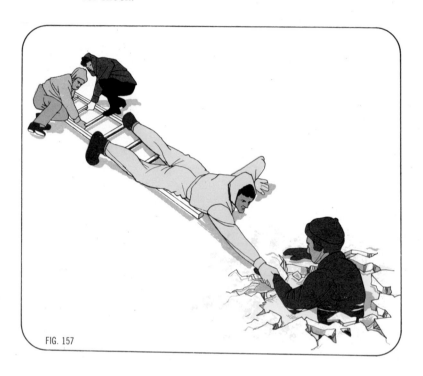

FIG. 157

INDEX